CONTENTS

1	Welcome
3	Prologue
5	Stage 1 - Introduction
10	Part 1 - My reason and my 'Why'
10	Chapter 1 - The Squashed Cabbage
15	Chapter 2 - Fear of a Short Drop
22	Chapter 3 - House of a Stranger
29	Chapter 4 - One Big Decision
38	Chapter 5 - Green Skin
44	Chapter 6 - My Biggest Failure
53	Part 2: The 5 Steps to Success
57	Step 1 - Part 1 - Honesty
59	Step 1 - Part 2 - Honesty
69	Step 2 - Priority
79	Step 3 - Fear
94	Step 4 - Ownership
103	Step 5 - Consistency
110	Muscle Up Your mindset
115	Part 3 - Moving Onto The Next Stage!

WELCOME

The 1st Stage in my 2 Stage process

I would firstly like to thank you for taking the time to purchase this book and take a break from your hectic schedule to spend some time with me, it really means a lot. I know we have probably never met, at most we have possibly exchanged an email or two, but I have had you in mind with each word I have included within this book. You are unique there is literally no one else on this planet like you. As much as this is true, we are all remarkably similar, we are all simply trying to path our way through life creating as much success and happiness for ourselves as possible. For many of us at certain points along this path we are knocked of by negative events or experiences which we find hard to overcome. The long-term effects of these experiences influence the actions and decisions we make in all aspects of our lives.

When I look at my son, I can't help but admire his innocence and simplistic view on life. He is not bothered by how he looks, what is going on in the world or how he is perceived by others, he's simply happy with some chocolate porridge and a cuddle. So at what point did we start making life complicated?

It is easy for us to get consumed by social pressures and lose focus on actually who we are as an individual. We spend far too much time conforming to social norms to gain Instagram followers or to get a complete stranger to double tap on our recent post.

Muscle Up your Mindset is a tool to reconnect you with you!

You will join me in experiencing some of the most memorable moments in my life and take away the lessons they have taught me. I will ask you to dig deep into your head space to find the real you and the desires you really want to achieve. After that all you need to do is take the lead and make a promise to yourself that from now on you are ready to commit and once again reconnect with you.

Yours Sincerely,
James Robertson

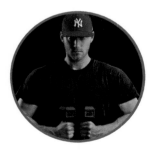

PROLOGUE

Hold yourself together James, I exhale deeply and turn to look at my brother in law for words of wisdom and reassurance. He looks at me and smiles, 'you ok mate' he says in a chirpy upbeat tone. 'Yes mate', I reply, I need you to do me a favour I said to him nervously, I need you to tell me when to turn around'. No worries mate, the bridal party are starting to come out now'. I stare up at the wooden beams supporting the top of the archway to the 16th century Keep known as the Leez Priory. I can feel the eyes of 101 guests burning into the back of my head. I feel an uncontrollable wave of emotion come over me as I fight back tears, hold yourself together I thought you can't cry in front of all these people, my eyes gaining focus on the wooden beams. My best man leans in, 'Albie's on his way down with Stacey's mum', I turn round to proudly see my 1 year old son walking down the aisle in his tiny black suit and white shirt, a very proud daddy moment for me as he looks so grown up with his strawberry blonde hair neatly gelled to one side. I exhale again and stare back up at the wooden beam as I focus on the weathered imperfections caused by such a long and distinguished history. 'James turn around now mate, Stacey's coming', I think to myself this is it, come on James this is the moment. I take a deep breath, exhale and then turn round, I look over a sea of people to lock eyes with my beautiful wife standing at the end of the aisle tears falling down her face as she tightly clutches the arm of her tearful father. I could not believe how beautiful she looked; the emotion started to build up, the guests turn to me sharply to gauge my reaction as I see my bride for the first time.

This moment was the proudest moment in my life and one I will never forget. For me it signified success, it was an indicator that I had made it in life and had been blessed with the most precious commodity anyone can have, a loving family of their own. The road to this point in my life was long and full of obstacles, I often wondered if I was ever going to become settled in life. At points I even thought life was never going to get any easier, and at times thought life had already given up on me. I want to take you on a short journey through some of the influential moments in my life, the moments that lead me to staring up at the wooden beams as I struggle to keep control of my emotions. The decisions we make in our present life are controlled and influenced by the experiences of our past. In order to ensure the decisions, we make every day are influenced from a positive mindset, we need to learn from past experiences, take on-board their lesson and move forward. Allowing the negative mindset to influence the decisions you make today leads you down an unstable and unpredictable road. By reading this book you have made a positive and proactive decision to allow the positive mindset to take the helm. With calm seas and a strong wind this book will give you a new positive outlook on life. You will begin your journey of achievement as you decide the outcome of the decisions you make every day. You will learn to enjoy the satisfaction you feel at the end of a hard day as you realise you have achieved everything you set out when you opened your eyes in the morning.

Right now I want you to fully embrace my mantra;

'You are a walking representation of your daily habits'.

STAGE 1

Introduction

The fact you are reading this is a huge step towards making change happen and I feel I have already learnt something about you. You are reading this as you are now committed to finally achieving your health, fitness and body confidence objectives that you have craved for so long to achieve. Well done you are arming yourself with the best battle armour ready to start this challenge.

So why have I taken the time to write this book as change happens in the gym and sitting on your butt reading this isn't changing anything? As much as this is true what you are doing right now is taking time to focus the mind and prepare yourself psychologically for a challenge in which success depends on just 1 thing, how psychologically resilient and focused you are, how much do you REALLY want to achieve this?? Before we begin any lifestyle change many of us wait for a burst of drive and determination to propel us over the first hurdle and on the road to success, this energy is known as motivation. But what is motivation other than a construct? Surely motivation is nothing more than a positive mindset, a mindset which is created by making little steps in the right direction, steps which when put together allows for positive changes to take place. All that stands in your way, laying in wait at the back of your mind is the lingering voice of negativity and its relentless attempts to keep you safe and protected within your comfort zone.

It is this voice which feeds you with doubt, encouraging you to question all those positive changes you are making, it tends to show itself in the form of excuses or idleness. But where does this negativity come from and how do you not only understand it, but learn to control it? Every decision we make in life no matter how big or small is influenced by 2 voices, the voice of negativity and the voice of positivity, which one you choose to listen to will determine the outcome of your decision and the direction of your life. All lifestyle change starts with the energetic determination known as motivation as you learn the 5 steps you need to take to develop a positive mindset and one which is focused and hungry for success.

Before we go into the details of how to Muscle Up your Mindset you need to commit! Right now, is where you decide to fully immerse yourself with the challenges that lie ahead, or stop reading accept you are not ready to face the challenge and continue on the path you are heading. If you are the latter then this is nothing to be ashamed about, each one of us is living their own life, with their own challenges and priorities. This book is yours now and if you are able to, take just one step forward commit to this book and as you read through we will start to understand each other and you will realise you are not taking on this journey alone, I am here supporting you every step of the way. If you are however battle ready and 110% committed, then I have just learnt something else about you, you are willing to step through the door I am presenting you with and slam it shut on your way through. You are able to grab an opportunity with a positive mindset and use this positivity as rocket fuel to success, for you success is simply a matter of time.

Part 1: My reason and my 'Why'

When I sit down with new clients and begin their consultation, I always ask them what it is they are looking to achieve. The common answer to this will be, 'I want to reduce my body fat and tone up'. This is great and highlights to me their desire for change in their life, we shall call this the 'effect'. As with all desire to create change there is often a deeper meaning, a deeper reason why the client feels that change is needed, so much so they are investing money into finding a faster and more effective method to achieve it. As a Personal Trainer and Online Coach it is my responsibility to make sure I generate the best possible result for my clients, and to achieve this I need to not only find a solution to the 'effect', but also allow the client to understand the reasons why they feel this change is needed, they need to understand their 'Why', this is known as the 'cause'. In order to fully gain control of the decisions you make every day and achieve a positive result it is important to learn the influencing lessons from your past and how they affect the outcome of your decisions today. Going through this process is how you learn how to 'Muscle Up your Mindset. So in part 1 I take you through some of the influential moments in my life, the moments which have made me the man I am right now. Our character today is a representation of our past experiences, it is vital that we learn their lesson so that they can positively influence our life in the future and the influencing decisions that we make.

Part 2: Motivation and the 5 Steps

In part 2 you start to enter the deeper parts of your mind, to be precise the amygdala and the limbic system, the parts of the brain that control your memory and your desire. You will start to understand the motivating forces which are influencing the decisions you make every day. It is these forces which are driving your desire to create change in your life, in part 2 you will start to understand your 'why'. Before making any change in our lives we all wait for this epiphany of motivation to lead us to success, but what is motivation and how do you become motivated? Learning how to manage and understand my own demons has allowed me to understand how to turn this negativity into a force of energy, energy which is used in all aspects of my life not just in the gym. By understanding your motivating factors, your allowing yourself to become intrinsically motivated, this is where you enjoy real success as the desire to achieve becomes just as important to you as the air you breath. Over time I have realised that I can develop a resilient and intrinsically motivated mindset towards any objective by going through what I have named the '5 Steps to Success'. These steps are Honesty, Priority, Fear, Ownership and Consistency. Going through this process will focus your mindset and turn any form of negativity into a force of energy which ultimately is going to power you through the door of the gym and on the road to success. This energy you could call intrinsic motivation. How we decide to view our world is determined by the challenges and experiences we have been exposed to in our life. These experiences develop your character, your mindset and your resilience as an individual.

Every one of us walks through life with 2 companions, the voice of positivity and the voice of negativity, both are there to guide and develop you in their own way. Which voice you decide to pay attention to is determined by the experiences and challenges we have faced from the moment we open our eyes. The voice of positivity formulates itself within your passions, your dreams and helps to guide you to be the person you want to be. Allowing this positivity to guide you will open your life to wonderful and fulfilling experiences. However, life is never so easy and is fort with danger and disappointment at every turn, exposure to this danger is unavoidable and is learnt from a young age. As a result, your body develops a natural shield protecting itself from this unavoidable danger, thus giving birth to the voice of negativity often presenting itself in forms of worry and anxiety. This voice is not your enemy it is there to protect you and keep you safe not only from danger, but from other evils such as embarrassment, failure and fear. Understanding the role each voice plays within your mindset is key to building resilience and focus, allowing either one to consume you will lead to nothing more than disappointment. By revisiting some of my earliest memories growing up I have been able to understand the lessons these experiences have taught me. I discovered how to understand my own mindset and the influence the 2 voices have on the decisions I make every day. It was through this journey that I released how to harness the energy from both and use them to keep me motivated and on a positive path. Right now I share with you some of my memories growing up and how they have guided me through my life right up until the moment I sat down to write this book. **So let's begin.....**

PART 1 - MY REASON AND MY 'WHY'

Chapter 1 - The squashed cabbage

I have a few memories growing up as a child, the detached house I grew up in, playing with my mates in the fields and only going home when the sun set or it was teatime. However, there was always a lingering aroma of negativity that never seemed to disappear, it would hang around like a grey cloud. Luckily as a child for the majority I was blissfully unaware of the reality of my surroundings and this was due to my mother who is an incredible woman and gave everything she had to me and my sister. I grew up in Lincolnshire in a small town called Deeping St James with my mother, father and sister who is 3 years older than me. Our town was small but friendly, you were never concerned about locking your front door or leaving your dog outside a shop. There were 3 churches, 1 supermarket and a river which ran all the way through. As a kid I would buy every single bag of Space Raiders I could and go fishing down the river with my mates. Although I didn't know it at the time, things for my family were tough and you could say we lived on the bread line. On a Sunday morning me and my mother would often walk to a local jumble sale in the townhall, she would spend hours rummaging through piles of second-hand clothes and would dust off old china items which she would use for the house. I still remember the mild smell of damp coming up from the bag of newly purchased items as we walked home.

A vivid memory I have is from when I was 8, my mother brought me my first brand new pair of trainers a black pair of Reeboks, as soon as I got home I opened the box and peeled of the white paper to put them on. Now to me those Reebok trainers could have been made of solid gold as I walked round the house so proud of myself. Looking out of the window it was a beautiful summers day and I remember my mother looking at me sternly saying 'your not wearing those outside', however being as proud as I was I didn't listen and ran straight outside into our lovely garden. Growing up our garden was beautiful with flower beds either side and 2 tall trees at the back which overlooked the playing field of the Primary School of which I used to go. Whilst I was playing with the hose pipe attempting to water the flower beds, I missed the plant and sprayed straight onto my left trainer. Now prior to this exact point in my short life I had never seen my mother react so furiously, I quickly removed the trainers and ran inside. My mother understandably outraged by my disregard of basic orders chased me round the house and threw the trainers at me whilst I ran up the stairs. Now I can hear my mothers reaction reading this memory right now as I always light heartedly remind her about it, and pretend this is the only memory I have from my childhood (of course its not I have many beautiful memories) but it is a stark reminder of just how tight things were growing up, and how her buying me them trainers probably meant that she went without for a while.

Food shopping was also a logistical nightmare, due to my father being the only driver in the house all travel was done on foot or on bike as it was very rare my father was home. For my mother this created a weekly challenge, how to get a whole weeks worth of food shopping from the supermarket back home with just a bike for travel and with a small child on the back. Looking back now one of my saddest memories I have was sitting strapped onto the back of my mothers old second-hand bike on a shopping trip to our local supermarket Rainbows. Her bike was white with a child seat on the back, dark brown rust covered the breaks and wheel rims due to years of weather exposure. We were about 5 minutes into our 20-minute bike ride home from the supermarket, me strapped in to the seat and the handle bar filled with between 6 to 8 shopping bags. While my mother courageously battled to steer the bike home, due to the friction from the tyre, one of the shopping bags completely split, the contents went everywhere! Vegetables and cans rolled into the road, I remember seeing the cabbage getting squashed under the tyre of a passing car. Due to the bike now being unstable we also went down with the shopping and hit the pavement with a cold thud. I don't remember being hurt myself but my mother clearly was however she never showed it. Whilst feeling seriously hurt and embarrassed she picked up what was left of the shopping and walked the bike home.

The lingering grey cloud I spoke about earlier was in the form of my father, growing up he was an unemployed alcoholic. He generally spent most of the money earned by my mothers child minding business on beer, resulting in little money for the family.

Every time he cut the grass, he would say to my mother that he needed to pop out to get petrol for the lawn mower only to come back 5 hours later drunk as a skunk. This sounds extremely negative and it was however many of my fondest memories were during these 5 hours when my father was out the house and those grey cloud disappeared for a short while. The three of us laughed and played in the garden, I was normally stuck up the tree or throwing marbles down the stairs.

Being a grown man with a family of my own I am now aware of her struggle back then and have no idea how she kept going day after day and remained positive for both me and my sister. This was my first experience of what true mental resilience looked like and it was in the form of a strong women protecting and raising her children, for that I will always be forever grateful. Mental resilience to me is the ability to look at a negative situation but to only focus on the positive elements which linger at arms reach, this is the only way to achieve a positive outcome from a negative environment. I learnt this early on in life when the grey cloud returned home. It was about 21:00 one evening and I was laying in bed looking up at my glow in the dark stars. I couldn't sleep for some reason maybe because past experience taught me that at some point my father would return, and this would undoubtedly result in arguments between my parents. I then heard the faint sound of a car pulling up on the drive and a key entering the lock to the front door, my father had returned with a gut full of beer, the arguments began and the doors slammed. I suppose this was my first experience of anxiety, that deep feeling of dread which would cling to the inner core of my body. I knew no harm would come to me and that I was safe in my warm bed, but it was the consistency of that anxious feeling that would slowly begin to fester over time.

Side note........

In the U.K it is reported that 1 in 6 people suffer with a mental health condition such as anxiety and depression. This statistic is based on those people that have reported concerns regarding their mental health directly to their G.P, so I imagine the real number is far higher. Guys this one is for you, lets be honest mental health is still a massive taboo amongst men, my father was a prime example of this. To my father any form of struggle was perceived to be nothing other than weakness and so he would struggle to show forms of emotion or talk to anyone about the negativity he had filling his mindset as a result of alcoholism to which he also strongly denied. As you progress through this book you will learn the dangers of allowing negative chatter to consume you and how important it is to pay attention to this chatter, understand it, and remember that it is simply just that, chatter. Anxiety is like a python, it can start by wrapping itself round your feet but before you know it, its wrapped around your entire body restricting your movement and ability to breath, its suffocating and just like a snake, can appear from nowhere. The negative chatter we all have every single day, about every decision we make is not the devil on your shoulder there simply to make your life hell, its your bodyguard and its there to protect you. The voice of negativity absorbs all the dangerous and negative information you are exposed to every day from the moment you are born, and it does all it can to protect you from it. The only problem is, this does not bode well with personal growth and development, as the simple concept of developing and growing as an individual means stepping outside of your comfort zone and into unknown waters. The positive voice says to open that door of opportunity, the negative voice says shut it, lock it and stay well away and so the battle goes on.

CHAPTER 2

Fear of a short drop

On a warm summers afternoon after I had returned home from school, I was around 14 years old and playing Frogger on our new Tiny Computer. My mother had sadly lost her father a few years previously and so we inherited a little bit of money, we also had a brand-new kitchen extension which was really cool. Whilst being fully engrossed in trying not to get the little frog run over, I heard my mother say 'James can we have a quick chat', she was stood behind me folding washing. I don't remember my mother ever asking to have a chat in such a soft and concerning manner so after the little frog got squashed, I turned round. I could see concern in her eyes like she was being crushed by an invisible weight, it was right now, this moment right now was the moment everything changed!

As soon as I took my hand of the computer mouse and turned around on our recently purchased office chair, my mother stopped folding washing and sat down at the dinning room table. As I watched her lips move and the words come out I knew that at no point in history has anything positive ever come from the following sentence, 'you know I love you, and that none of this is your fault'. That anxious feeling that I remember gripping me as a child when I was lying in bed, it returned and I sat there feeling like my insides were being squeezed from within, at this point my mother got straight to the point. I suppose there is no good way to deliver bad news, so she just came out with it, 'me and your father are getting divorced'.

I understand that divorce happens, and it is a sad reality for many families with hundreds of children going through the turmoil of hearing such news every day. In this situation the best outcome is that both parents act maturely and amicably for the sake of the children, to come to a resolve and move forward. In the worst case scenario, neither parent leaves the marital home, one parent meets a new partner and the family home becomes a boiling pot of emotion and tension, yes as you already guessed my situation was the latter. One fateful afternoon my mother was on the drive with her new partner, as they kissed to say goodbye my father returned home from work. For some reason that day he decided not to go to the pub after work and as a result all 3 found themselves stood on the driveway to the family home. To make things worse not only was my father an alcoholic but by this point he was also a Prison Officer at a Category A prison. Alcohol, a furious temper and your Ex standing in front of you with her new partner does not make for a tasty cocktail. Now weirdly the details of this event are vague, maybe this is my brains way of protecting me psychologically or maybe I just didn't want to remember. All I do remember was everyone erupting, the time for diplomacy was over, I remember feeling worried that my mother was going to get it from both sides so I grabbed her, holding her arms behind her back while she struggled to break free. She was shouting at me to let her go, only so she could throw years of emotional turmoil straight in my father's direction. I remember shouting in her ear 'you're not going to beat me for strength, so stop struggling!' She eventually accepted this and when everything calmed down, I let her go. My mum wanted my Dads throat that day as my fathers reaction was far from diplomatic.

I seem to recall him pulling out his prison batten, a long wooden bat, like a rounders bat with a solid led core. My father used to think it was hilarious to walk past me in the house and use the bat to tap me on any accessible bone he could, I can confirm that even a little tap with that bat in the right place hurts like hell. I can understand the reaction of both my parents that day. For my father, seeing my mother with her new partner was the final confirmation that his marriage was over. I think deep down he hoped that things would blow over and return to normal, this confirmed to him my mother was serious. The sight of them together hit my dad hard, no one likes to see their Ex with their new partner especially your wife of 20+ years. For my mother however that moment on the driveway was a final drop in a very full cup, after years and years of psychological turmoil, although she was an incredibly resilient person, proved too much.

The days following the driveway incident were intense to say the least, emotions were flying high and the house was like a boiling pot! My father when not at work or down the pub would just sit in the kitchen with a glass of whisky in one hand and a cigar in the other. As he dabbed his cigar into an old wooden ash tray made from the hull of a sunken 19th century Naval Ship, I could see a very broken man, there was no emotion behind those eyes it was like he was made of steel. Someone said to me once that your eyes are the window to your soul, and I strongly believe this. Your eyes can tell you a lot about a person, revealing inward emotions that the individual is trying hard to conceal. I attempted many times to start a conversation with him in an attempt to gain any evidence I could that my father was still present and that he had not been completely lost to a deep dark pit of depression.

Looking back now at this point my father was a broken man and probably suffering from depression but he would never admit this. My father was a stubborn man who did not suffer fools lightly, he would portray no sign of struggle of any form as this would be nothing more than pathetic weakness in his eyes and as a man this was not acceptable, he was seriously old school. When I was younger my father would say to my mother that she babied me too much, and that I was going to grow up gay because I used to tell my mother that I loved her. I used to tell my mother that I was thankful for all the kind things she did for me. I remember thanking my mother once by just randomly coming out with, 'mum, thank you for looking after my life', I suppose this shows the kind person my mother had brought me up to be.

Life at home was becoming fragile, the negativity and depression which had completely engulfed my father was like a thick black smoke that when breathed in would grab hold of your sanity and absorb it like water to a sponge. It was becoming infectious and between me and my sister I had taken to it the hardest, the black smoke of negativity seeping into my bloodstream. This negativity was starting to consume me turning a once loving and compassionate boy into cold stone. This was where the battle with my demons began and it is still being fought today. By this point things were looking dire, my father's drinking had increased to a seriously unhealthy level. My mother was getting ever closer to my now step dad and was even staying round his house to get away from the family home, which by now had thick black smoke of negativity oozing out of the open windows.

Although I didn't know it back then, my step dad really is a top bloke and since the dust settled on this turmoil period of all our lives, he has been the only real positive male role model and mentor I have had in my life. I now see Keith as my real father and for that I am incredibly lucky.

At some point something or someone was going to crack, there was no way you could keep this level of tension boiling. Then one evening everything came to blows, the temperature that had been ever increasing had blown the lid off the boiling point pot that had been the family home, we had all cracked! The night previously I had walked into the house to find my mother round my step dads house and my father sat on the sofa with his head in his hands. He was full on crying, as mentioned earlier this does not happen, I did not even know my father had the ability to cry. After walking into the house and seeing my dad, I sat down on the sofa and put my arm round him, at the age of 14 it felt strange to be in a position of role reversal but the sight of my father crying had hit a nerve. I remember him saying to me that he had no other option, he had nowhere to go and the only option he had was to go the same way as his mother who had sadly committed suicide a few years earlier when I was just a boy. Holy Shit I thought! What am I supposed to do now? By now tears were falling through his tightly squeezed fingers as his grip became tighter and tighter around his head. I hopelessly attempted to try and remind him of all the positivity he had in his life in an attempt to control the negative chatter completely invading his sanity, but I'm not going to lie there wasn't much and we both knew it.

I said to him that no matter what decision he made I would go with him, even if it meant he lived in the caravan we brought a few years earlier from my mother's inheritance money, I would go with him. After probably the toughest 10 minutes of my life that tough, hardened exterior of my father started to return as he began to get a grip of the negativity that had taken over him. This took strength and was the first time I had seen someone pull themselves out of what was probably a mental break down to form a more reasoned and logical mindset. However that night I had breathed in the thick black smoke of negativity that surrounded my father and just knowing the possibility that my father was going to kill himself was enough to make deep cracks in my vastly crumbling sole.

Side note.....

When it comes to success in life never underestimate the power of a positive mindset. To gain control you must train your mind to become stronger than your emotions, if you don't you will lose yourself every time you hear negative chatter. If you begin this journey with any doubt or negativity regarding your ability to achieve success, the voice of negativity will start to seep into your mindset and influence any positive decisions you make. This is exactly why 50% of new members to the gym throw in the towel and leave after just 6 months. The voice of negativity tells them that they don't have time for the gym and that there are more important priorities that need to be addressed. Right now, it seems people are far more insecure with their bodies than at any other time in history and there is a very simply reason for this. The modern world accepts nothing other than perfection and will openly criticise anything that is less than perfect.

The phrase 'dadbod' only come about in 1994 by American student referring to the typical body shape of the middle age man. For all the dads out there we all know that when a child comes into the world the last concern on your list of priorities is your appearance and that is exactly how it should be, but this doesn't stop the world trying to convince you that it's not acceptable. When it comes to having a baby those who really pull the short straw are all the incredible mums out there, how you physically build a human whilst going through your daily life astounds me. One of the best days of my life was the day my little boy was born as my wife Stacey courageously brought Albie into the world.

Bringing a child into the world is the most amazing spectacle, but so many new mums soon start feeling the pressure that their bodies should bounce right back to how it was before they were pregnant, which is crazy when you see what they have been through. You see female Fitness Influencers posting pictures of how quickly they managed to get back to shape after giving birth, but doesn't this highlight that sadly to that individual being visually perfect to the world is more important than spending time with their new baby, I suppose this just hits the nail on the head with modern day expectations. If the excuse is that you have no time for exercise, then this simply means that your success in the gym is not a priority or at least sitting in your top 5. Peoples priority lists will change all the time and that's life we are all travelling at 1000 mph, literally and at that speed the outcome of those changes depend on how much you pay attention to the quiet voice of positivity which lingers at the back of your mind.

CHAPTER 3

House of a stranger

The evening that followed my fathers shocking revelation that he was considering suicide was equally as concerning. For some reason again I remember little of this evening just the key events. It is interesting that my memory is vague during the most traumatic events at least for me. I was sat at the top of the stairs of our family home and remember seeing my mother at the foot of the stairs with her new partner, after yet another argument surrounding my father and in a fit of anger she informed me that both her and my new step father were moving to Spain to get away from everyone and the horrendous situation we all found ourselves in. I don't blame her we all wanted out, but I had no choice but to stay immersed in the turmoil, I was only 14. This was the final drop in a very full glass for me, I completedly emotionally crumbled. In the last 24 hours I learnt my dad wanted to kill himself, my mum was moving to Spain, and I was just getting ready to start my GCSEs. I remember sitting on my bedroom floor an emotional wreck with no idea where to turn or what to do. All I remember from this situation was my father saying that enough was enough he was finally moving out, the sight of his son a mess on his bedroom floor finally triggered a logical response from him! On hearing this, I immediately knew 2 things, 1. The pressure was going to ease slightly in the family home which was going to be good for everyone. 2. I had no choice but to move out with him, if he was to tie a dressing gown cord round his neck id never forgive myself for not being there to stop him.

The next few days passed reasonably peacefully, luckily my mother never did move to Spain, the statement was simply a release of anger and frustration due to the situation. Learning that my father had finally agreed to move out, allowed my mother to finally breathe a sigh of relief. After months of slowly boiling in the pressure cooker that was the family home my mother could finally get her home back and release the thick black smoke of negativity through the open windows. Luckily, my mother was in charge of finding my father a new place to live, if it was down to him a mattress next to the depressed goldfish in his local pub would have sufficed. A couple of weeks later she found my fathers new home, a lovely 2 bed house just 10-minute bike ride from the current family home. So, a couple of days later while my mother was at work, my dad hired a van and we both moved all our possessions into our new bachelor pad down the road. I remember feeling overly excited about this and spent days planning our new house with my father while he sat in the kitchen with a cigar in one hand and a glass of whisky in the other. I was mainly excited as I had never moved to a new house before and this literally felt like I was moving out to live with a mate. Moving day came and I spent ages sorting out my little shoe box room that would just about accommodate a single bed and a wardrobe. I even got to have a TV/VCR combo and a phone in my room which was pukka, I could literally lay in bed on the phone whilst watching Black Hawk Down for the 13th time a film that would have a greater impact on my life than I knew at the time. Things finally relaxed a little and my dad even seemed in better spirits. On the other side however me moving out had hit my mum HARD! She knew that I was talking about moving out with my dad, but she didn't think I would actually do it.

She had no idea that we were moving out that day, my father did this deliberately so that he could just go hassle free without any more driveway incidents. After work she walked in the front door, expecting to see me sat on the computer or watching TV, nothing! She went upstairs walked into my room to see a completely empty bedroom, all that was left were the glow in the dark stars on the ceiling and an empty skeleton of a wardrobe. My mothers heart sank, as far as she was concerned, she had just lost her son! All the turmoil and pain that she went through to raise me while my father drank away our money, and I'd thrown it all in her face and abandoned her for the man who was the route cause of our hardship growing up. This hit my mother so hard it would take a few years for her to come to terms with my decision that day. At this point however she had no idea of the conversation I'd had with my father during that night of turmoil. She was unaware that I made the decision to move out purely due to the fear that my father was going to kill himself. As far as she knew I was done with her and had thrown the previous 14 years back in her face.

Peace with my father didn't last long, the emotional pain he was trying so hard to hide started to surface and this was for one reason, he was back in the pub and drinking more than ever. I soon realised the novelty of moving out to live with my father had worn away and the grim reality of my situation revealed itself. I was starting to get used to waking up in the morning to an empty house as my father was at work, and going to bed in an empty house as he was down the pub, I was 80% self-sufficient at the age of 15, I even used to do the food shopping. I started missing the love and comfort you would expect from a family home and used to lay in bed thinking about all the happy times I'd had with my mum and sister growing up as a child. Two weeks had passed since I made the decision to move out of the family home, I had not even spoke to my mum on the phone. The absence was simply to allow me to get my head around my new life and to try and silence the ever increasing 'negative chatter' that was in my head. For my mother however it was confirmation that I was gone without even saying goodbye. I started to miss my mother more and more each day and craved the loving support that you need at such a young age. So, one evening while my father was at work, I made the decision to go back to the family home and see my mother, I needed her.

I didn't know what to expect from my surprise visit, the last I had seen her was the day before we moved as she was up early for a 6:30am start that day. I turned up to the front of the house and walked across the block paved driveway towards the door. This was the house I had spent my entire life in, but right now it felt like a stranger's house. I did not expect to feel this anxious about returning home, but that gut-wrenching feeling returned. I suppose this was because deep down I knew that me making the decision that day to move out and abandon my mother was out of order, she did not deserve to walk in to see an empty room that day. After a couple of deep breaths on the doorstep I walked in. I found my mother in the kitchen doing the washing up, on hearing the door opening she peered over her shoulder, through the corner of her eye she saw me stood in the hallway looking anxious and like a complete stranger. She has never spoken about how she felt at this moment seeing me after 2 weeks but her body language spoke a thousand words. The reception I received was a very cold one and looking back now I can understand why.

She had spent the previous 2 weeks going over and over in her head about what she had done wrong to drive me out of the house, especially after spending the last 14 years giving up everything for me and my sister. She was suffering but at the time I didn't know this, all I knew was she had changed, she didn't want to know me. On looking over her shoulder, she paused acknowledge the fact I was stood there and carried on washing up. I do not remember anything else from this moment, I guess what stuck with me was the nervous, anxious feeling I felt returning home after 2 weeks and the stranger I found in the kitchen. I knew I desperately needed my mother, as living with my father was tough and emotionally I was struggling. Deep down I was starting to realise that the relationship between me and my mother was never going to be the same again, this time I had cut too deep.

This life became the new norm for me at least for a while, living on my own for much of the time while my dad was down the pub. I remember feeling nervous as I sat in anticipation just waiting for his return, not knowing if he was going to come home depressed or looking for a fight. As a result of this emotional battering, I started going round to see my mother more and more. The more I went round there the more comforting and welcoming it became and I started to realise that my step dad was actually a really nice man, he brought out a positive side to my mother that I'd never seen until now. Before long I did not want to leave, the thought of going back to my father's house used to fill me with dread and anxiety. However, I had made my choice and that was now my home, so I had a decision to make, mentally toughen up or emotionally crumble. Now subconsciously I decided to toughen up and had a simple but effective method for silencing the increasing negative chatter that filled my head. Without purposely doing so I would find myself looking at my reflection in the mirror whilst brushing my teeth silently asking, 'what the hell is wrong with you?', 'why do you feel like stone', 'what are you doing with yourself'. It would be during these conversations with myself in the mirror that I would process all the anger that I was feeling at that point and try to rationalise everything into a more positive mindset.

Side note.....

We all experience negativity every day, some more than others and this is ok, it is here to test you. Negativity comes in all shapes and sizes; we are subjected to continuous negativity through the media such as the news. Womens magazines are literally covered with stories about a negative situation someone has been in but are still here to tell the story. As a society we have a strange relationship with negativity, we hate it and find it difficult to deal with, but yet are fascinated with how other people who have experienced a negative event in their life managed to deal with it. How you dealt with this negativity determines not only the outcome, but also your resilience and development as a person, do you become consumed by it? Or understand that it is there, but filter the information to allow for it to be positively processed. My father always used to refer to a negative situation with the phrase, 'just call it character building'. This phrase has always stuck with me because it is an amazingly effective way of looking at negativity. It suggests that you understand that negativity is just chatter, you positively process it and allow the driving seat of mindset to be driven by the voice of positivity.

When it comes to making positive changes to your life you potentially open yourself up to criticism. As a society we love to pick faults with each other, someones body shape, how much they earn, what they do with their spare time etc, we are all subjected to this negativity every day. But the real reason for this is because not only do we love picking faults with people, but we also hate any form of success that is not our own. As soon as someone starts to make positive changes to their life, whether that be a job promotion, getting fit or losing weight people hate it! They hate it because it highlights their own lack of achievement and drive to be successful. You are starting to achieve the rewards that they desire but they are not in a positive mindset powerful enough to achieve it. They are consumed by the voice of negativity which is keeping them pinned down within their safe zone. I am making you aware of this as you may experience this form of negativity as you start to grow, change and develop your body and mind through the training you are about to begin. People will become threatened by this and start to turn what is an incredibly positive change, into something negative and can be perceived as being selfish. But you are strong enough to deal with such chatter! You understand that such chatter is simply the words of a person held down in life by the voice of negativity. The most powerful achievement you could make from this situation is to achieve all you set out to and develop that positive mind and body so much so that not only have you changed your life, but you are now also influencing this person to break free from the negative chains which hold them back. You are now a role model and an inspiration, and no achievement can give you more internal pride and a feeling of accomplishment.

CHAPTER 4

One big decision

This is where my life took a turn, and you could say it was this moment right now that has had the biggest impact on my life and career today. I knew I had to create an outlet for the anger I felt burning inside and desperately needed to conquer the negative chatter in my mind and the insecurities I had with my body. I decided to set up a gym in my fathers garage, by throwing away a lot of the left over items from the house move I managed to create a big enough space for some basic kit, I thought to myself where is the best place to buy gym equipment, of course there was only 1 choice. I pulled out the Argos catalogue and started sifting through their fitness section, I did not really have a clue what I was looking at so stuck with what I recognised from PE classes at school. My new fitness studio had within it a bench press, 1 barbell, 2 dumbbells and a heavy fabric punch bag donated to me by my sisters boyfriend. Being over 6ft and weighing around 11 stone I was a bread stick in shorts, and I'd had enough! Weight training became my stress relief, it became my medicine and in my head the solution to all my problems. I haven't mentioned much about this so far in my story but on top of all the drama I was getting at home, I was also getting a hard time at school being bullied on a daily basis by older lads, probably because I was taller and younger than they were making me an easy target. However again I had an easy solution to focus that negative energy, I drew the faces of the 4 main lads I was getting grief from onto my punch bag, each face also had its own speech bubble with a hateful comment they would typically say.

This helped me focus and to gather up all that hate and anger that was boiling inside and unleash it all into that punch bag not stopping until I was knackered or blood was pouring from my bare knuckles. This method of therapy worked and not only was I starting to get a hold of my crumbling mental state, but I was also starting to become fitter and physically stronger. Right now, was the first time I discovered the power of exercise both physically and mentally. I started to do research into weight training and would watch videos on YouTube in the evening. A big upcoming company at the time was called 'MaxiMuscle' and they were everywhere, believing all the adverts I had seen I also purchased some weight gain protein powder and started drinking it daily to help me build some muscle. I knew I looked like a bread stick and this made me an easy target for bullies, but I was determined to change that as I saw this as being a major weakness, I thought that if I could muscle up my body it to would muscle up my mindset. I suppose that mindset has never really left me, even now when I am in a situation where I feel uncomfortable, I become withdrawn and think to myself I wish I was bigger, I'd feel safe and confident right now if I was. I even felt like this when I was 18 stone of pure muscle and buying T-shirts was impossible. The lesson learnt here is you can change your body but this doesn't mean it will solve any insecurities you have, they tend to become ingrained into your mindset and are hard to shift, I have however learnt to control this negative chatter. The lessons I learnt during this period of my life have lead me to be the man I am today with a beautiful family of my own and a career which allows me to change the lives of so many people and it all started as an angry kid in his dads garage.

Everything in my life was starting to fall into place, I was seeing my mother and stepfather every day and the relationship was building with my mother as we began healing those deep cracks that were caused a couple of years previously. We also managed to have the conversation about the real reason why I moved out and the emotional damage that day had on us both, we still occasionally talk about it today when I take my family over to see them. They brought a lovely house together just outside my village in a town called Langtoft, a lovely 4-bedroom detached house with a gravel driveway leading up to the front door with a little wooden dog on the doorstep. There was a beautiful garden with a low-level fence overlooking multiple fields of corn and cabbages, it wasn't long before I started to crave this peaceful and idyllic environment.

My father had also started seeing a new partner a lady named Lindy and before long she moved in which was great. I now no longer felt any guilt about leaving my father on his own, this guilt used to haunt me as I was ever fearful that if left alone he would drink too much and do something stupid, however with his new partner supporting him I knew he was safe. She was a funny character about the same age as my dad, weirdly I remembered her from Scout camp as a child as she used to be a Scout leader for a different unit, she had bushy grey hair and looked a little like Charlie Dimmock from Ground Force. She always seemed to be in the garden or cooking food which obviously my father loved. Over time I started to see that kind and funny side to my dad return which for years had been drowning inside due to depression and alcohol abuse.

What I still find hard to come to terms with today is the fact that had my father been like that all the time, he would of made a fantastic father and husband and the story I am telling you now would have been very different, I suppose that is the grim reality of alcoholism. I would pop over to see him and find him watching TV on a weekend or out in the garden potting plants, the days of him either being at work or in the pub had gone. Seeing him so happy lifted an enormous amount of pressure from my shoulders, pressure which had been pinning me to the ground for so long, this finally allowed me to make one big change in my life. I moved back in with my mother and stepfather to the idyllic home in Langtoft, now finally I had a safe and supportive family home.

A few months passed and I was making regular trips over to see my father and his new partner, normally she'd cook something like a warm hearty bolognaise and leave it on top of the cooker ready for me. I would walk in the front door and see a happy smiling man sat on the kitchen worktop with a cigar in one hand and a glass of orange juice in the other, you could almost say he had finally changed. I would then hear that phrase that will never leave me, 'alright Jay, hows things?'. Now to most people this is a very common question that when asked, you probably wouldn't really register it as the automatic response would be 'yeah not bad mate'. But to me my father asking me this question in a happy joyful voice reassured me that he was doing ok and that finally he had found some happiness. One day I popped over and decided to check out my old garage gym to see if everything was still there. The punch bag was still hanging there, the dry stale blood still covering the faded faces I'd drawn onto the canvas.

The bench press I'd pushed so hard on for so long was now covered in bags of old clothes and knitting from when my fathers partner had moved in. As weird as it sounds, when I looked into the garage that day, the place which not so long ago was filled with the blood, sweat and negativity of that troubled time, had also found peace amongst the flowery bags and half knitted jumpers. I was 16 now and despite all the instability over the previous 2 years I had still managed to leave school with 8 GCSEs from A* to C which despite everything is an achievement I am proud off. Looking back now the decision I made to toughen up emotionally as oppose to crumbling into a state of depression is how I managed to successfully pull myself through that period of my life. The conversations I used to have with myself in the mirror almost daily combined with my ability to off load my stress and anger in my garage gym, focused my mindset and kept me going. It wasn't until recently when I started to look back at this period of my life, that I realised I had not only managed to muscle up my body but that I had also successfully Muscled up My Mindset, this is ultimately what has lead me to this point in my life today. If you learn to harness the power of a focused mindset, you can open doors which at the time feel as if they are locked shut forever, but only by opening doors will new and exciting possibilities be presented.

My new peaceful and hassle-free life did not last for too long as my father had once again hit rocky ground, so I popped over to see him one afternoon after he had finished work. I put my key in the lock to his front door and walked in, I received the happy, 'Alright Jay how's things' it was a positive start.

My father was still holding onto that new chirpy demeanour which found him some happiness, he also had a glass of orange juice in his hand however, the house was quiet, noticeably quiet. Where's Lindy I asked. 'Ahhh I threw her out my dad replied in a funny manner, 'Ooook' I replied, 'Any reason?'.

Now the following sentence which was about to leave my fathers lips is probably the weirdest comment anyone has ever said to me. 'Yeah she kept stealing my shoes and giving them to homeless people'. I couldn't help but laugh at the fact some homeless men are sat in a bus stop in Peterborough smoking crack wearing an extremely well polished pair of standard issue prison boots, they were so buffed you could see your reflection in the toecap. It turns out once a week Lindy was working in soup kitchens in Peterborough and whilst my father was at work, she would steal a pair of his shoes and hand them out along with a cup of warm soup. This was bad news, although my father still appeared to be in a positive mindset, this would not last long as now he was left unsupervised with just his fragile mindset to keep him company.

Life continued very much as it was for some months, I would try to make regular trips over to see my father. This became slightly harder as time went on as the regular trips to the pub after work returned and the glass of orange juice I used to see him with when I popped over, was soon replaced by what looked like apple juice, until I sniffed it. One evening I popped over to see my father, I rode my bike over to his house and put it in the garage.

I was 17 and had recently received my provisional driving license and had begun the driving lessons bought for me by my mother and step father for my 17 birthday. I turned up to find an empty house, he was off work and so that only meant one thing. I called him to find out he was down a different pub than usual, it was outside of the village and was too far to ride my bike to, however after a quick call to a friend I was dropped of at the front door. I walked in to the familiar sight of my father propping up the bar with a pint of fizzing bubbles in front of him. He seemed in good spirits but with a few pints of Stella flowing through you blood stream you would be.

After engaging in small talk for around 30 minutes my father finished his beer, picked up his keys and said come on lets go home. As he walked towards the door I realised that he was actually planning on driving home and to say he was over the limit would be an understatement. 'Your not driving home', I said to him forcefully, 'If you get pulled over your lose your job'. 'Alright' my dad replied as he threw me the keys, 'You drive'. Now this was a situation I really didn't want to be in, if my father drove and gets pulled he's finished and unemployed. If I drive and get pulled over, I could lose my license before I even got it. I quickly completed a risk assessment in my head and decided the outcome of my father getting pulled would be far worse, so I got into the driving seat of his blue Ford Scorpio, the smell of cigar smoke clinging to the upholstery.

I pulled out of the pub and turned left towards the bypass, my father decided he was 18 again, he cracked the radio up to full blast, opened the window and stuck his head right out.

While his head was bouncing around like a Labrador, as loud as he could he started singing 'All along the Watch Tower' by Jimmy Hendricks while air guitaring inside the car, we were a police officers quarter pounder with cheese. We got onto the bypass, Jimmy Hendricks still banging on my ear drum, when my father pulled his head back into the car, 'go faster' he said forcefully, 'go faster, you want to learn how to drive go faster'. Before I knew it I was doing 100 mph down the bypass with my dads head hanging out the window howling like a dog. I was shitting it! After a 10 minute drive which normally would be 20, we pulled into a housing estate and I had an excuse to turn the music down and drive like a civilised person, before long I pulled onto my fathers drive. To say I was relieved was an understatement. However seeing my fathers reckless behaviour that night did highlight my already lingering concern, my father had retuned back to his old negative mindset of which was only suppressed through alcohol.

Side note.....

Before starting any form of fitness journey many people seem to wait for the 'epiphany' of energy known as motivation to suddenly appear, filling them with energy and powering them through the door to the gym and on the road to success. But this never happens! So does motivation really exist? Or is it simply the accumulation of little positive steps encouraging you into a more positive and motivated mindset. These little steps usually begin with an episode of honesty, the sudden realisation that you are not happy and that there needs to be change. Motivation does not exist when a sudden required desire for change is not present. This means that you can harness the power of motivation and it all starts with being brutally honest with yourself.

I realised this during the mirror sessions I had when I was 14 and living with my father. I would wake up in the morning and while brushing my teeth, be brutally honest with myself about what I was, who I was and what I was becoming. This brutal honesty allowed me to understand where I was in my life and the direction in which I was going, at the time it was not a good one. Failing to be brutally honest with yourself can allow you to be clouded and standing in the shadows of your reality. It is easy to perceive yourself in a way which may differ from the truth, as it is much easier to be in denial than to face your true reality.

Real change in your life can only happen when you are able to look yourself in the mirror and be brutally honest to yourself about your flaws and your desires. Only once you move passed this stage are you able to move forward and develop a positive mindset powerful enough to create change, this is what motivation is! Once you move passed this stage, your newly formed inner energy can be activated by simple triggers.

Now that you have faced the honesty mirror, you are in the right mindset to use this energy to build yourself back up, focusing on your desires and your newly formed positive mindset. Now that you know the areas of your life you need to work on, simple triggers can release this inner energy to motivate you to complete the task. This could be something as simple as watching a training video on YouTube before going to the gym, or looking at previous pictures and reminding yourself why you are focused on achieving that outcome. Success will only come after a compelling moment of honesty!

CHAPTER 5

Green Skin

After the Jimmy Hendricks cruise we thankfully arrived onto my fathers driveway in one piece. He opened the car door and stumbled towards the front door with a very confused look on his face. With his right hand in his pocket, he rummaged around desperately trying to find his keys in the belief that he had just simply driven home from the pub. He was completely oblivious to the fact I was stood there with the keys in my hand after driving him home like Fast and the Furious. That evening after my father went to bed, I laid staring up at my bedroom ceiling with the sickening realisation of one fact, all the turmoil and negativity which had engulfed my father for all those years had returned. A negative mindset is like your shadow, black in colour and can suddenly appear from nowhere, and just like your shadow will always be there lying, waiting to appear. I could feel the shadow of negativity creeping into my mindset as I felt the dreaded concern overwhelm me, my fathers safety was now going to be my sole responsibility, again. I needed out! But this time, permanently.

I was starting to lose the new positive mindset that had kept me focused through my GCSEs and into a better mind space. The muscled up mindset that was originally powered through my moments of brutal honesty in the mirror and the intense garage workouts which left my knuckles bleeding, was starting to fade, being replaced by the negative chatter of worry and doubt. I couldn't lose this I couldn't surrender to the negativity that was filling my thoughts.

After a few nights of staring up at the ceiling, I tried to put together a positive plan of action to get my life back on track, these sleepless nights lead me to making one of the biggest decisions of my life, I'm going to join the Army. I had been trying for over a year to join the Army as to me it meant structure and purpose, I would know the direction I was going in my life and my responsibilities would be laid before me. However, this was halted by one major issue, as a child I'd had asthma and to pass Army selection you were required to be 4 years clear from the last date you were issued an inhaler. I still had another year to go! But this did not stop me from pursuing the possibility of finding a loophole, and after a couple of months of investigation incredibly I managed to find one. It was during a conversation with my doctor regarding my plan to join the Army and the fact it was my medical background holding me back that lead him to do me a massive favour. He wrote me a letter free of charge stating that I had formally been clear of asthma for over 4 years and was cleared to continue with selection, this was all I needed, I could finally apply. The following day after celebrating with my mother, I took the bus into Peterborough and walked proudly into the careers office. While I was sat there waiting for a member of staff to assist me, I was reading a leaflet all about the Royal Engineers and it sounded right up my street, you get a trade, you learn to become a soldier and you also get to blow stuff up. I was sold! I was going to become a Sapper. I completed the application form and arranged the first stages of selection. When you apply to join any branch of the Armed Forces you are required to pass what's known as 'Selection' for me this was a 3 day course at the Glencorse barracks in Scotland which was currently home to the Black Watch a Scottish Infantry Regiment, seriously hard men.

After 3 days of intense testing I managed to pass with an A Grade which meant I would begin training on the next intake, I was finally in the British Army! I was awarded my pass certificate on the day which I was to take back to the careers office so they could arrange for me to attend my Basic Training. I was pleased as punch and held that certificate the entire 4-hour train journey back to Peterborough. This was to date the proudest moment of my life and I felt despite all the odds and my medical struggles to even apply, I had made it. Finally, my life was on track and my outlook and mindset was full of positivity. I had silenced the negative chatter that had consumed me for so long, I had put it in a box and locked it tight. I was certain that from that moment the box was never going to be opened again, I had won the battle.

A few weeks later after a lot of physical training, my bags were packed, and I was sat in the back of my stepfathers car as we drove towards the train station once again. My Basic Training was being held in a town called Lichfield which is near Birmingham, it was where most Royal Engineers begin their training. As I sat in the back of the car that day my head was a whirlwind of emotion, I knew from that day my life was never going to be the same, I knew that I was walking into the unknown, and I was walking on my own. As we stepped onto the platform I could see my mother was trying hard not to show how she was truly feeling as she fought hard to swallow her emotions. She was trying hard to stay strong in an attempt to help me remain positive, little did she know I was doing exactly the same. I said my goodbyes and gave my stepfather a firm handshake, the kind of handshake that lets you know your safe and that everything is going to be ok.

As I stepped onto the train with my bag full of gear, I looked up at them both as they stood on the bridge looking over, a tear running down my mothers face. It was right now that the negative chatter crept back in and began polluting my mind. I began to question my decision and if I had really made the right choice. This is natural however, don't forget negative chatter is there to protect you and to keep you safe in your comfort zone, I didn't know what the hell I was walking into and this meant the voice of negativity was very present and very loud. I tried hard not to let this chatter consume me and focused hard on the adventure I was about to embark on and the doors of opportunity this was going to open. The train was extremely busy and so in a corner by the door, I sat on top of my bag leaned back and cracked open a can of coke. I took a deep breath in and the voice of positivity said, ' right buddy, here we go, its time'.

Side note....

Negativity is like a parasite, sucking the blood and energy out of your body every day and just like a parasite you may not even know it is there unless you start paying attention to it. Understanding negativity is the key to turning this parasite into a positive energy which will focus the mind and drive you through the door to the gym on every workout time after time. When you start paying attention to negativity you start to recognise just how often the voice of negativity tries to influence the decisions you have to make every day. Once you start paying attention to this voice you will start to recognise that there are similarities within the way in which the voice attempts to influence you. The voice of negativity will always show the follow characteristics:

1. It will always take the easiest available route around a decision which often steers you away from producing a positive outcome. When it comes to getting in shape the voice of negativity may attempt to keep you at home and safe on the sofa by telling you exactly what you want to hear. You don't need to go to the gym to get rid of that unwanted body fat and that this can simply be achieved by following a fad, calorie restricting diet. You know deep down that this is not true and that exercise is a vital component in achieving a toned and confident physique, however the voice of negativity is clever and knows exactly how to keep you in your safe zone and sat at home.

2. The voice will always try to justify its influence on you by giving examples in which it knows you will pay attention to. When it comes to the gym, these are the excuses you have buzzing around your mind convincing you that a better option would be to stay at home. The two most common statements you will hear are, 'I don't have time for the gym' of course you do have time we have 24 hour gyms everywhere, however you have been influenced to spend that available time doing non productive activities which keep you safe at home on the sofa. 'I'm too tired', the truth is very few people have ever experienced what true tiredness is. What most people feel is a slight temporary change in the regular physical and mental challenges of their day to day life creating an urge to rest. Don't be fooled into thinking this is genuine tiredness, it isn't! Your body is capable of producing so much more and is able to adapt easily to this new requirement for energy.

3.   The voice will always respond to a negative situation with negativity. When the voice of negativity is at the helm of your mindset it will be almost impossible to find a positive resolve to the issues you face every day. Your default reaction to a negative situation will be to immediately defend yourself and your actions, potentially pushing blame in a different direction. Fighting a negative situation with negativity will only produce one result, a negative one. This brings us to one of the 5 steps of a positive mindset, 'Ownership', you need to take ownership of your daily actions and decisions, then use this information to produce a positive outcome. This is tough and requires a level of understanding of your own mindset, and the triggers which cause the voice of negativity to begin influencing your decisions . This is where you start to realise exactly what it is that fuels the voice of negativity, its your emotions. Once you realise this you will be able to predict exactly when the voice of negativity will raise its ugly head and begin to manipulate your mindset and your decision-making abilities. Negative emotions such as anger, jealousy, anxiety, disgust and fear will always feed the voice of negativity to influence you into responding to a situation negatively. Understanding this means you will be ready for the voice of negativity to attempt its manipulation, but you understand that by listening to this influence will only result in a negative outcome. You have learnt that this voice is nothing other than chatter and that when ignored allows for positive outcomes to develop.

CHAPTER 6

My biggest failure

The train came to a steady stop and the loud 'beep beep beep' could be heard as the doors began to open, I had arrived at Lichfield train station. I picked up my bag, threw it over my shoulder and stepped onto the platform. As I scanned the station signs for the exit route I started to notice other lads a similar age to me walking towards the exit with a big bag and a shaved head, at least I'm not on my own I thought, those lads must be with me. As I walked outside the station there was a small gathering of lads all with the same confused look on their faces. They were a mixed bunch some tall, some short, some with big mop hairstyles and others with shaved heads we all came from totally different parts of the country and had totally different backgrounds. But we all had one thing in common, we were wearing a suit for the second time and had no idea what the hell we were doing or what we were walking into. A bus pulled up and stopped right in front of us, off stepped a soldier in his green camo uniform and a clipboard in his left hand. We were all made to stand in a horizontal line facing the bus with our hands behind our back. By observing his uniform I could see that he had achieved the rank of Corporal however he stated that we were to refer to him as 'Staff'. He began to read of a register and one by one the lads confirmed their attendance. We all piled onto the bus and the normal social bantering began between the lads. I sat there quietly looking out of the window as I fought hard to keep the negative chatter at bay.

But no matter how hard I tried the negative emotions of anxiety and fear crept into my mindset I was nervous as hell! Shortly the bus arrived at the training Barracks and I could see troops of soldiers on the parade square all at different stages of their training, I remember just looking at one troop in particular with pure envy that they had almost finished their training and were about to go home. We exited the bus and began to make our way to our accommodation block. We all stood to attention along the corridor as the directing Staff directed us into each room. A standard accommodation block for the Army is a large room divided into 3 parts each with 6 beds in each section. Each bed had 2 wardrobes, one for uniform and kit and the other for civilian clothing or 'Civis' as they were known. Each bed also had 2 cupboards across the top for extra kit storage. We all knew that we were going to get to know each other pretty well over the next few weeks as we slept, showered and trained together and so the normal questions began between the lads, how old they were, where they were from, what they did before they joined the army and how they had all given their girlfriend a hard leaving present before they left, the normal peacocking behaviour amongst lads. However was struggling inside the voice of negativity was 100% at the helm of my mindset and the emotions I was feeling were far from positive. This confused me as I had waited for so long to join the Army as I saw it as the answer to all my problems. With the voice of negativity at the helm, as far as I was aware, I did not want to be there. Once we squared all our kit away, I had to attend registration and attest into the British Army. We queued up outside a dark building, which was poorly lit by 3 lights hanging off the ceiling.

At the end were 3 more directing staff, all in their standard Army Uniform sitting behind a table. They were confirming the trainees name and chosen trade which they would move onto once they had completed Phase 1 of Army training. After queueing for a while I was called up and stood to attention in front of one of the tables, 'Name' he stated, 'Sapper Robertson' I replied. 'So your going to be a Plant Operator are you', Yes Staff' I replied 'it was the only trade available'. He looked up at me, 'So you like digging graves then do you'. I paused in silence as I processed what he had just told me, 'Next' he then said loudly as I turned and made my way out of the building. A fucking grave digger I thought, that sounds proper shit. I really didn't need to hear that as I was already battling hard to keep myself focused. Later that evening when we had a little down time to square all our kit away, I popped outside and gave my mother a phone call. She asked the normal inquisitive questions, ' how is it?', 'whats it like?', before I had even given her an answer a surge of emotion came over me, I had been completely consumed by the anxiety and fear which was infiltrating my mindset, I cried, for the first time since my father said he wanted to commit suicide, I cried.

There is one particular phrase I heard recently, 'You have to train your mind to be stronger than your emotions, or you will lose yourself every time', looking back now this phrase could not be more relevant as I had allowed my emotions to take full control of me. The next day we all woke and made our way down to the scoff house for breakfast. Our first task for the day was to pass a second medical examination before we could begin the physical challenge of Basic Army Training. Before I had attended the training school it was very common for me to get pains in my right knee, this was mainly due to playing so much sport as a child and at times would result in me limping of the rugby pitch. I knew this in the back of my mind however before attending Lichfield when I was in a positive mindset I said to myself I would just get on with it and try to ignore any pain that presented itself. However while I was waiting outside the Drs consultation room I was far from being in a positive mindset. I was called in by the Dr for examination, I was passing all the tests with flying colours until the Dr asked me one question, 'do you have any underlying injuries which may prevent you from training'. Now the voice of positivity was in the back of my mind whispering, 'say no and carry on', but that voice was quickly silenced by the negativity that consumed me. I informed the doctor of my knee issue and was quickly taken to see a physiotherapist for further investigation. Later that day it was concluded I was unfit for training and would return home to rest and return on the next intake 6 weeks later. The first thought that came into my mind, 'what the hell have you just done'. Immediately after I received this news, I rushed down to speak to one of the directing staff pleading for a second test, however it was too late the paperwork had been processed. Just before I turned to walk out of the door, he stopped and said, 'don't worry too much Robertson, we will see you in 6 weeks', well that's something at least I thought, but I knew I had royally fucked up.

As a result of my imminent transfer out of the Lichfield Training centre I was placed in a new troop 'the loser bin' as it was known as the whole troop was made up of individuals who for different reasons were awaiting a transfer out. My departure would take a few days to sort out due to all required paperwork and transport passes.

This meant we were marched around the training centre to complete different tasks most of which meant hanging around in our accommodation waiting for the next mealtime. Occasionally we passed our intake of recruits as they began their training, I remember marching passed them one morning as they left for PT (Physical Training) I watched them as they run off in their tight formation, I knew full well that if id kept my mouth shut chances are id be leading that run by now. The day came for me and 3 others to leave the training centre, we were given our discharge papers and a free train card home. The bus pulled up to take us back to Lichfield station, the place I had arrived at ready to start my Military career a mere 5 days previously. I was gutted and even pleaded again with one of the directing staff to allow me to stay. The only element of positivity I was hanging on to was the fact that the corporal informed me I was to return to my careers office back in Peterborough and book myself onto the next intake in 6 weeks time. I spent the next 2 hours on that train sat with my head in my hands wondering how the hell I was going to face my family after they had waved me off just days before.

After arriving home with the heavy burden of shame weighing me down, I picked myself up yet again and marched down to my local careers office the very next day to arrange for my next intake. I had to get back there, I had to prove to myself and my family that I was not a failure. I arrived and stood in front of the tall glass building and pressed the buzzer. A friendly female voice asked me which branch of the armed forces I was here to see and allowed me in. I sat in that waiting room my heart in my mouth as the negative chatter played over and over in my head, 'what if I cant get back in', 'what am I going to tell everyone' my stomach started cramping with anticipation.

To take my mind of the tension I picked up a brochure on the glass table in front and started reading about different Infantry regiments in the South East, to be honest this sounded far more interesting than digging graves . As I got halfway through, a figure appeared down the hall way in the standard green uniform of the Army, 'back again so soon he said' it was my careers officer, he walked me through to a private room and sat me down, I explained what happened and he pulled out my file. Time stood still as he flicked through the folder, I informed him what the Corporal had told me, and that I was here to be booked onto the next intake. He looked up from the file with a concerned look on his face, 'you have been medically discharged' he said 'what does that mean I replied quickly?', 'it means you're out, there's nothing I can do' instead of arranging for me to attend the next intake I was MD from the Armed Forces, was it an admin error or was the Corporal wrong? Either way it was irrelevant, I was out of the British Army before I had even started. My heart sank, my worst nightmare had come true and what would have been an opportunity of a lifetime had been thrown away like a bag of rubbish. I had screwed up, worse than that I had failed not only myself but my whole family. I drove back home, walked straight up the stairs, and sat on my bed with my head in my hands. Up until this exact moment in my life I had been through mental challenges but I had never felt the internal disappointment of failure, and I only had myself to blame.

Side note....

Failure is one of the hardest psychologically emotions to process as it is confirmation that we are not perfect and that we know there is going to be judgement placed upon us by all those that we are close to.

Failure has the ability to instantly change our mindset as the voice of negativity punishes you over and over again, reminding you of your faults and convincing you that you do not have the ability to achieve your dreams. This constant self-destruction can easily take you to a very, very dark place as it continuously knocks you down. The problem with failure is not only do you have to suffer the internal battering you are giving yourself, but you also have to battle the judgement from others as they ask probing questions such as, 'So what happened then', 'Why are you back so soon did you fail?' and then my worst question, 'So what are you going to do now? Despite the constant negative chatter and internal battering, you are giving yourself there is still an element of positivity which can be pulled from this pit of darkness. We are all human and failure is a part of life, we are all going to fail at some stage in our life. I knew that I had to get a grip of my mindset and this meant I had to understand two key factors. 1. I have to take full responsibility for the failure. 2. It was only me who could get myself out of this hole of self-pity and on the road to something more positive.

The best way to deal with failure is to look upon it as a life lesson, review what went wrong to cause the failure and make sure this never happens again. It is easy to allow yourself to remain in this dark pit of negativity and sadly for many this is the long term result of failure as they struggle to get a grip of their mindset and rationalise the outcome into something more positive and manageable. Failure is a sign that you have stepped outside of your comfort zone, to fail simply means that you have attempted to grow as a person and develop yourself however the challenge was too large at the time. People who have never experienced the feeling of failure have probably never attempted to step into the unknown and grow as an individual. Failure is nothing more than a pat on the back and a voice saying, 'never mind, it's happened, pick yourself up, next time we know what we are doing'. Being able to look upon my failure more positively took a long time as I could have easily looked at myself as a victim and blamed the Army for an admin issue which had placed me in this position, but that was never going to change the situation I found myself in, I needed to take responsibility. This was not the end of my service in the Army, as months later I had passed my selection course once again and found myself on my way to Catterick to start my infantry training as part of the Princess of Wales Royal Regiment PWRR. This time I was mentally ready for the challenge and instead of feeling gripped by anxiety like I had previously, I enjoyed every minute of it and thrived in the challenges presented. The truth is, if I had not failed at that moment in my life I would not be where I am today with the family and experiences I have been able to enjoy, including a University degree which has placed me on the path I follow today. That moment of failure was a pivotal moment in my life and one which has had a positive outcome. If you view failure with a positive mindset only a positive outcome can be achieved, the same goes for a negative mindset, the decision is yours.

Essex is the LA of the UK!

So we have reached the part of my life which saw me quite randomly ending up in Essex. I heard a saying once that Essex was the LA of the UK and so after leaving the Army with large ambitions to set myself up as a Personal Trainer I thought that sounded like the right place to start.

I packed my bags on the 24th January 2012 threw them into the back of my blue 1999 Honda Accord and punched SS3 into my sat nav. I had no idea where I was going or what I was going to do but entering the unknown this time was exciting, I guess this comes with life experience. Over 8 years later and I am sat here writing this book with over a 100 successfully trained clients under my belt and ready to launch my brand-new online brand. I have never stopped enjoying the challenges presented to me every day and can safely say I love my job and the life I have built. I must say the last 8 years have been interesting to say the least, I could write a book on the experiences of a Personal Trainer and would be confident that it would sell, maybe this could be my next project!

Until then all I will say is, I have no longer regretted any decisions I have made and look forward into the future with excitement and ambition, I want this for you. Thank you for joining me through the first 30 years of my life and going through some of my most profound memories. I have taken you on this journey to show you that the positivity and direction of your life is 100% in your control and only you have the power to create change. It all starts with a small step and the fact you are reading this book before you begin your new health and fitness challenge, tells me you are already on the right path. This is exciting and I can't wait to see what is waiting for you when you reach your destination. Right now you have got work to do, you have been through my journey and now it's time to create yours, its time to learn the 5 steps required to Muscle Up your Mindset....

PART 2

The 5 Steps to Success

By reading through part 1 of this book and experiencing some of the most influential moments in my life, you know that I have been presented with a variety of both mental and physical challenges. I look back at these challenges now through a positive mindset and understand that they were there simply to test me and prepare me for all the challenges that present themselves in the future. I want you to look back at challenges you have faced in your life with the same positive mindset and understand that it has been these challenges that have made you the person you are today. It is easy to play the victim card and allow your past to mould who you are today. However, this is never going to allow for the positive outcome you deserve, understanding this is the first step to Muscling Up your Mindset. When I was thinking of a name for this book I tried to look back for moments of inspiration, moments that changed my life and guided me onto the path of positivity. The truth is, there was not any such moment, you are in full control of your own destiny no matter what challenge is presented to you. Before you can change the positivity of your environment you need to take ownership of all challenges presented, they are yours and yours only. By accepting this you are now able to decide if the outcome from this challenge is going to be positive or negative. I first discovered this living with my father and trying to get my head around the psychological effect this environment was having upon me, I was quickly slipping into a very dark place of violence and self-destruction. The only reason this changed was because I confronted myself in the mirror and faced the demons staring back at me. All negativity needs a positive outlet, allowing negative emotions such as anger to fester in your mind results in the negative mindset taking full control of you. Remember if you allow your emotions to control your mindset, you will lose control every time. I found this positive outlet within my garage gym, the workouts allowing me to focus the anger I had building up inside and overtime I was able to process it and gain back control, for then at least I was winning the battle. It was this form of therapy that cleared my mind and allowed me to think with clarity and focus. Through this process I not only muscled up my body but also my mindset and so there it was, the perfect name to describe my story and the lessons I have learnt.

Fitness saved me in several different ways, it has been this lesson that I have tried to share with others throughout my career. To help influence people and ultimately allow them to live freely has been the focus of my career. The role of a Personal Trainer is to help their clients live without the burden of negativity and able to look forward in life with a positive outlook, confident that they can finally attain the body they desire. To achieve this, I use the '5 Steps to Success', these steps have pulled me through not only dark times but also times where I feel I face a mental barrier.

I still use this system today during times when I need to take a step back from a situation and take a deep breath. Please feel free to use this method to help you in any aspect of your life and I hope the 5 Steps allow you to make positive and decisive changes. As fitness has had such a positive influence in my life, I will be using the process to show you how adopting a healthier lifestyle can achieve a similar outcome for you. The 5 Step process will be used to ensure you keep a positive mindset and allow yourself to remain focused on not just the results, but also the journey you are about to go through. As mentioned at the start of this book 50% of people who attend the gym drop out within the first 6 months. This is because they are allowing themselves to be influenced by the voice of negativity, keeping them firmly stuck within their safe zone. They never get a firm grip on the challenge fat loss brings and as a result push blame for this failure on other aspects of life, such as work commitments and relationships, justifying this failure with the excuse, ' I don't have time'. As you now know all challenges you face in your life are yours, take ownership of them and take control of the outcome. Small steps in the right direction, lead you on the path to success.

I want you to close your eyes and picture yourself standing next to an empty swimming pool, with your swimming costume on and your towel in your hand. You investigate the swimming pool with disappointment as you can see the shiny tiles on the dry base of the pool.

Now, you have a choice;

You could accept the pool is empty, walk away and carry on your life with the disappointment that you never got to experience the joy and pleasure the water would have given you.

Or

You can take the positive approach and start to fill the pool one bucket at a time, knowing that eventually you will be able to dive into the cool and refreshing water enjoying the end result of all your hard work.

Right now you are staring into that empty pool, at the beginning of your journey battling in your head about whether you are in the right mindset to make the lifestyle changes required to finally achieve your body composition goals. Remember, every workout you do throws a bucket of water into the pool, every day you manage your calorie intake you throw a bucket of water into the pool. It is only a matter of time before you are diving in head first and enjoying the refreshing water. Take full responsibility of the challenge ahead, embrace it, pick up your bucket and let's begin......

STEP 1 - PART 1

Honesty

Before you can make any positive changes to your life you need to be completely honest with yourself about who you really are. Being honest with yourself is an extremely difficult process to go through but is vital to allow you to move forward. Living a dishonest life full of smoke and mirrors means you are not only being dishonest with those around you but also with yourself, this will never allow you to reach your full potential and live with integrity. The honesty stage will begin with you coming face to face with yourself in the mirror. No-one else knows the truth about the person staring back at you other than you. All those skeletons you have laying at the back of your mind will be confronted face to face, pull them out of the cupboard and confront them. These skeletons are the subconscious influences effecting the outcome of every action and decision you make every day. To focus your mind into a positive outlook you need to face these demons, understand why they are there, learn their lesson and then bury them. These demons need to be processed to prevent the voice of negativity from using them to influence you further and damage any positive outcomes in your life. A moment of honesty is also required to allow you to see the flaws which are holding you back. If your lazy tell yourself that, if you tend to give up as soon as something becomes hard, then be honest, you need to lay out your flaws. This process will be achieved over time, the more time you spend confronting your flaws, the easier it will become.

The more flaws and demons you lay bare in front of you the easier it will be, as they are steadily processed, they will become less and less. By laying your flaws in front of you, you are allowing yourself to understand your weaknesses, once you take responsibility of these weaknesses you can control them. When you face any type of challenge in your life the voice of negativity will attempt to use these flaws to influence your actions, decisions and ultimately the outcome. If one of your flaws is your lazy, the negative voice will tell you to stay at home and not go to the gym. Unless you understand that this negative chatter is simply exploiting your flaws to influence your decision and keep you in your safe zone, you may well listen to it. You are now fully prepared for this as you have confronted these flaws one to one. You will see this attempt to exploit your weaknesses straight away and understand that the influencing voice of negativity is simply just chatter, nothing else. You will ignore this influence and in fact by doing the complete opposite will result in a positive outcome. Right now, you are taking full control of your mindset and your emotions, using them as a form of energy to achieve the task in hand and push you through the door to the gym and throwing another bucket of water into that pool. You will battle the negative chatter every day, once you have learned to ignore it, you will start to hear the positive whispers at the back of your mind, focus on those and a positive outcome is all that will be achieved. Once you have been through this process, you will have confronted your demons, processed them, and then buried them. You should feel a big heavy weight lift off your shoulders, enjoy this feeling, you have now been through the hardest stage, well done. Now you are ready to allow for positive influences to take hold, you are ready to take on the next stage of honesty.

STEP 1 - PART 2

Honesty

Ask yourself the following question, 'what do you want to achieve?'. This question can relate to anything you want to achieve a promotion at work, to achieve a better work life balance or simply to lose weight. For the sake of this book we are going to focus on the latter although the process will work for any challenge you wish to conquer. So, you want to reduce your body fat and get back into shape? I am guessing this is also not the first time and you have previously attempted this challenge several times before and achieved no long-term success. First of all don't be too hard on yourself, you were not armed with the knowledge required to complete the task successfully and were I'm sure influenced by industry 'gurus' who were leading you down the wrong path simply to make some money. Sadly, a high percentage of the fitness industry is made up of such 'gurus' who feel they are in a position of expertise simply after completing a 6-week course at a local college. You can normally spot these 'gurus' as they will attempt to catch your attention on social media with a picture of them topless whilst advertising their quick fix diet approach, or plugging their ambassadorship with some supplement company selling a solution to all your problems in a pill or drink form. Avoid these people at all costs, they are exploiting your vulnerability and insecurities just simply to make money, trust me when I say your results are not their main priority.

Just as a side note, if a diet has a name or a time frame, for example 'take the low carbohydrate diet and see dramatic results in just 6 week' do not follow it, diets such as these create results through dramatic and unsustainable calorie deficits. You will see results short term however due to their unsustainability it is just a matter of time before the weight comes back on, you will be back to square one after learning absolutely nothing, the only thing that is lighter is your bank balance. Short term diets create only short-term results. To finally achieve sustainable long-term fat loss, you will need to learn to enjoy the journey, the lifestyle changes and all the benefits that come with them. We will cover this in further detail within my 'Progress Tracker', where I go into more detail around all variables effecting fat loss and what is required to be successful.

I want you to ask yourself another question, 'Why do you want to achieve this?'. Setting yourself challenges and objectives to achieve daily, weekly and monthly is exactly the proactive approach which leads to personal growth and development, but it's always a good idea to dig a little deeper and find out exactly why you want to achieve this certain objective. If your objective is to improve your work/life balance, then by digging a little deeper you may see that the reason for this is to improve your relationship with your family. You may feel as though you are not giving enough time to your children due to the stress and pressures of your job and this is the real reason why you need the lifestyle change. In this example your family then become your motivation to succeed, your desire and need to spend more time with your children becomes your energy and motivation to make sure this objective is successfully achieved.

In Honesty Part 1 I asked you to be honest about who you are as a person, to face your demons and understand your flaws. This was to allow you to gain control over your mindset and recognise when the voice of negativity attempts to influence you by using your flaws as ammunition. Remember, if your mindset is governed by your emotions you will fail every time, so it is important you are in full control. By looking a little deeper into the real reasons why you want to achieve this objective, you allow yourself to fully embrace the benefits that will come by achieving success. When looking at weight loss for example, if the only reason you want to lose a bit of weight is to achieve instant gratification through your pictures on social media, then this maybe hiding a bigger issue that simply won't be resolved by losing a little bit of body fat. Please understand that confidence is only increased by fully embracing the journey, making life changes, adopting a more active lifestyle and by successfully achieving your goals. Therefore a quick fix diet will never truly give you the results and happiness you truly crave deep down. So why do you want to lose weight? Once you have the answer to this question you are fully armed with the fuel that will drive you on the road to success.

The difference between intrinsic and extrinsic motivation.

Before we start any form of lifestyle change many people like to wait for the epiphany of motivation to energise this change and create more proactive behaviour. But what is motivation, and does it really exist? Google says that 'motivation' is the process that initiates, guides and maintains goal-orientated behaviours'.

So, by this definition, if you were to be 'motivated' you would able to start your journey, guide yourself through the challenge, achieve the result and then maintain these results long term. Now as I mentioned earlier I am going to assume that this is not your first attempt at achieving successful long term fat loss, so based on the above, can we then assume that you failed previously simply because you were not correctly motivated? So how do you become 'motivated'? There are said to be 2 types of motivation and these are the Google definitions of both:

1. Intrinsic motivation: Is the act of doing something without any obvious external reward. You do it because its enjoyable and interesting, rather than because of an outside incentive or pressure to do it.

2. Extrinsic motivation: Is reward driven behaviour, rewards or other incentives like praise, fame or money are used as motivation for specific activities. Unlike Intrinsic motivation, extrinsic is driven by external factors.

If we look back to the original definition of 'motivation' you can clearly see that one of the characteristics is the fact you guide yourself through the challenge and sustain long term results. This would then suggest that the reason so many people fail to achieve long term fat loss results is simply because they are extrinsically motivated, they are driven by the attention and gratification they receive from other people by achieving these results. I see this every day and the fitness industry I am sad to say is probably one of the leading contributors to causing this huge decrease in peoples self-esteem and confidence.

Therefore, people are going to social streams to gain the attention and acceptance they crave. When we scroll through social media for example, it is only a matter of seconds before we start coming across people showing of their flawless and seemingly perfect bodies. In fact, we see so much of this material every day that it has now become the norm and young people especially now, feel pressured to look exactly the same, perfectly flawless with no imperfections. Now here is the grim reality of the fitness industry influencers that are setting this standard. They are lying to you! They have not achieved their physique by following their own diet and training plans! This standard is impossible to achieve unless you do exactly what they do and a high percentage of Instagram influencers achieved these perfect physiques by doing the following, this relates to both male and female influencers:

1.   Take steroids

2.   Spend 2-3 hours per day in the gym, they do not have full time jobs so are able to do this.

3.   By making themselves and their physique the only concern they have to worry about every day, family and friends come second.

4.   They spend the rest of their day stressing out and worrying about their food, preparing it, cooking it, and moaning about it.

How do I know this? Because this used to be me!

So the very industry people are turning to in order to achieve this extrinsic motivation and gain the guidance they need to achieve a flawless physique, are lying to you straight away and setting an impossible standard to hit for any teenager or adult who has a full time job and a family to look after. No wonder the UK health and fitness industry has a market worth of around £5 billion, with 20% growth in the last 5 years alone. What would be a seriously alarming statistic is how much of this income was generated as a result of insecurities caused by social media! Extrinsic motivation has a noticeably short time frame, the attention and gratification that is received by achieving such results eventually slows down, the number of new followers starts to decrease and so does the number of post likes. The sad thing is today a persons success and popularity is based purely on how many followers they have on social media and how many LIKES they can generate on a single post. If this is the motivation behind your objectives, then you are setting yourself up to fail. Not only that but negative emotions such as anger, anxiety and fear will take full control of your mindset as the attention starts to disappear and no matter how much fat you've lost, you will still feel disappointed and alone. You may have achieved the objective, but the reasons for the need to achieve this objective were external and so you were never going to fully enjoy the achievement. As we look deeper into the epiphany known as motivation we start to find possible reasons why so many fail to achieve the results they are after, it would appear this is simply down to the fact they are motivated by the wrong external forces. They focus more on the response they will gain from other people by reducing their body fat as opposed to achieving the objective for positive reasons such as an improvement in their confidence, self-esteem, and overall happiness.

The attention they gain from others will at some point start to fade, and as this is the main force driving their motivation so will the desire to continue, this will result in relapse and steady weight gain. Sound familiar? We shall call this process Yo-yo dieting. If a person is intrinsically motivated to achieve an objective then they are driven every day by the most powerful of all the motivating forces, pride! A person motivated through pride is not interested in superficial gratification such as popularity or feels the need to adhere to social pressures. They do what they do every day because of the joy their daily habits bring them both mentally and physically. A prideful person is powered every day by a positive mindset, they take ownership of all challenges presented to them. It is by conquering these challenges that fills them with pride and motivates them onto the next challenge. So, what is the definition of 'pride':

According to Google, the definition of pride is: 'A feeling of deep pleasure or satisfaction derived from ones own achievements, the achievements of those with whom one is closely associated or from qualities or possessions that are widely admired'.

When we look at the definition of both pride and intrinsic motivation, we can start to see similarities between the two psychological characteristics. An intrinsic person carries out their daily tasks due to the enjoyment they bring to their life every day. These tasks all start with making your bed in the morning, this sounds easy but be honest, when you are in a rush in the morning how tempting is it to just leave your bed a mess and crack on with breakfast? If you fail to make your bed after you fall out of it you are already starting your day off by failing your first task.

Use this opportunity to enjoy a little win first thing, if you don't your starting off the day negatively and this mindset will continue. It is through the successful completion of these tasks that overtime creates positive results no matter how large or small. You will seriously appreciate that made bed when you fall into it after a hard day at work. Take social media for example, a Personal Trainer can schedule 30 minutes a day to post meaningful content, when they look at the engagement they receive on one particular post it might be quite low. But despite the lack of instant gratification from these posts, it is through the consistent completion of this simple task every day that over time builds a following which over time turns into clients and ultimately sales. If a person was extrinsically motivated to complete this task chances are they would have been put off at the first few posts due to the lack of the instant engagement and gratification they were hoping for. It is this sense of achievement which overtime turns into pride. The Personal Trainer understands that the financial reward has been achieved purely through their hard work and commitment to the daily tasks, this resulted in client leads, and a lump dropped into their bank account. A prideful person thrives on conquering challenges every day and enjoying the success that this brings. However, as a society we hate success, well other peoples success at least. For some reason people are easily offended by a successful person, simply because it highlights that individuals lack of success and motivation to conquer their daily challenges. As you can see being motivated by pride is a very powerful emotion, and one that can drive your behaviour every day. So why is it when you type 'prideful person' into Google the results are so negative?

Here's some of the statements that are presented on page one of Google when you search 'prideful person';

* *A prideful person is arrogant and doesn't have many friends.*

* *A prideful person has a hard time accepting failures.*

* *They are often offended when their behaviour is questioned.*

* *A prideful person believes they have it all figured out, so they don't need to listen to an expert.*

I find all this negativity quite sad but it simply shows the mindset of the majority of people in society. Most people are offended by a prideful person simply because they are not affected by the social pressure to be like everybody else. Negative people are offended by a prideful and positive person because they highlight all the flaws a negative person has. We are a society that hates success, to the point where we slate it. A negative person will do all they can to put down someone who has achieved any degree of success, because it highlights their own failures and lack of achievement. They will say things like, ' I don't know what they have done to deserve that, I work far harder'. They will see your achievement like it is something you won; they will be offended because they feel they deserve to have what you have achieved. But you have what they do not, a positive mindset which is powered simply by internal pride. Do not be the grey man, be proud of who you are and what you have achieved. Be the shepherd not the sheep!

So I ask you again, 'Why do you want to achieve this?' Hopefully now you can see that this question is bigger than you probably first thought. You might be that individual right now that appears to be externally motivated and that is fine. All this simply means is that you have not looked deep enough into your soul, you have not spent enough time in the mirror facing your demons and taking ownership of your flaws. Try and find the reason why you are craving instant gratification from people and why you feel the only way to achieve this is to change your appearance, what has caused this lack of confidence in you? This is the question you need to ask. As I mentioned earlier you will live a far happier life when you become the shepherd, just simply be you and learn to love the person you are. Trying to be the sheep and conforming to the opinions and beliefs of how others think you should be, is only going to create a negative mindset as you are putting yourself into a position where you cannot win. You are not being true to yourself, and the gratification you are craving from others, you're never going to receive because don't forget people hate success and so by achieving your objective is only going to create a negative response. People will only praise your success when it appears you have not been as successful as them, as soon as you pass them, they will start to resent you, simply through jealousy. So, who are you doing this for you, or them? Please never change who you are to please other people, the only person you can be is you, and your perfect there is no one else on this planet like you, your unique.

STEP 2

Priority

Chances are you are sat reading this book because up until right now you haven't made yourself a priority and as a result are drifting further and further away from the person you were and the person you feel you should be. You could be a loving husband and family man doing all you can to provide for your family and give them the best you can. You could be fully immersed in your career that you have no time for yourself and so each day rolls on and on, before you know it the person you see in the mirror is a stranger. But don't worry you have been through the honesty stage of this book and that was not easy. You are now fully in control of your mindset and have been honest about who you are now, who you want to be and the reasons why you want to achieve this, all you have to do now is change your priority list.

I mentioned earlier that a huge 50% of people who have attempted to successfully reduce their body fat and change their physique, fail and cancelled their gym membership after just 6 months. Now through the Honesty stage we discovered that this may be due to the fact they were motivated by external factors, and this is probably true. But if you speak to these people after they have handed in their membership cancellation a huge 60% say the reason is that they simply do not have time. I can't help but think that this is simply an easy excuse to bypass the question. We have 24 hour gyms so having no time simply cannot be a genuine reason for giving up on one of your desires.

One of the beautiful things about life is the variety of challenges we are faced with every day it's what makes life interesting and keeps us driven towards success. Each challenge will come with its own positives and negatives. As we know by reading through this book the mindset we approach each challenge with will influence the outcome that occurs. Every day we are consciously and subconsciously placing all these daily challenges into a priority list, as I mentioned earlier the first challenge we face every day is making our bed and we do this to start the day in a positive mindset. Now each person walking this earth is unique and is carrying with them the heavy weight of their priority list and the stress that comes with it. Although everyone is different, I am a strong believer in the saying, ' you can never judge a man until you have walked a mile in his shoes' basically meaning, you never know the challenges that people face every day and the tasks that sit at the top of their list, so don't judge them. Society norms dictate that for the majority of us our priority lists are going to be very similar. I would imagine that for a high % of the population the top 3 on their daily priority list would look something like this:

1.   Family – the need to provide for them and keep them safe.

2.   Work – to build a solid career which allows you to achieve number 1.

3.   Daily chores cooking food, tidying the house and doing the washing.

These will obviously vary slightly depending on if you have children, a career you are passionate about and have a house to look after, but I would image many will relate.

As you can see the top three objectives on our daily priority list cover the majority of the stress and worry that we battle every day, they are important and so any issues relating to them cannot be simply ignored.

Before we carry on with this book, I want you to write down what your top 5 priorities are every day. This may seem hard to start with, but if you dig deep enough you will find your 5, they are 100% lurking in your Hippocampus somewhere (Hippocampus is the part of the brain where memories are formed). I'll give you a couple of minutes.

Now looking at your top 5 priorities, can you see your fat loss goals on your list? If not, why not? I know what your going to say, 'but James you don't understand I literally don't have time, I have 3 kids, a cat, a goldfish and a husband to look after as well as a full-time job'. I get it, I'm also a father to a beautiful boy and know that the moment you become a parent your priorities change. I went from a full time Personal Trainer who occasionally carried out some fitness modelling and stood on stage in his pants during a physique competition, to walking up and down the landing at 2am trying to get a tiny burp from my little bundle of wind, for the third time already that night. The fact remains, your body is not going to credit you with an easier fat loss journey due to your external commitments. The decision to create change is 100% down to you, if you don't make the mindset switch and start to prioritise yourself no one will. I would like to think though that this mindset is starting to switch a little through reading this book, after all it is called Muscle Up your Mindset.

If your fat loss goals are not at least number 5 on your list, I think you need to re do your list and rethink your priorities. If achieving your fat loss goals is really that important to you. Attempting a fat loss challenge when in your own mind you're not committed to it, is like getting dressed up for a job interview for a job you don't even want, but you still go to the interview anyway. Nothing positive is going to come from this, your going to end up exactly where you are now but with the bitter disappointment of yet another failed attempt. In the 'Honesty' part of this book we looked at the different forms of motivation and their effects on your mindset. We learnt that to be successful your drive needs to come from intrinsic pride as opposed to extrinsic determination such as instant gratification. But what if I was going to tell you that your primary motivator depends entirely on your priority list. If reducing your body fat sat on the number 2 spot on your list then you would do everything you could that day to make sure it was achieved, just like you do for work which is currently number 2 on our hypothetical list. Your whole day would be based around what was required to achieve the task to the best of your ability. You would make sure you hit your calorie and protein targets, that you were burning as many NEAT calories as you could through daily movement and that your sleep and hydration were on point. The reason you do not, is simply because your brain is full of other daily challenges which for you, sit higher on your priority list. Moving your fat loss goals up to within your top 5 and making the mindset switch to becoming more focused on you, is exactly what the phrase Muscle Up your Mindset is all about.

Are you making time for you?

Since becoming a father my life has dramatically changed and it does from the moment your baby is placed into your arms, that urge to protect, love and nurture that baby tops all other stresses and priorities you have in your life. The day my son Albie was born was the best day off my life and one I will never forget. He came as a surprise on 4/5/2018, arriving 5 weeks early whilst my wife Stacey was in the middle of her work baby shower, she even turned up to the maternity ward wearing her pink 'MUM TO BE' sash, what a geek. One of the biggest changes that occur when you become a parent is the fact you are no longer your main priority, you can't be, its natures way of ensuring you do all you can to love and protect your baby. Overtime this constant neglect both physically and mentally will start to take its toll on you. All the late nights, poor diet and high stress levels will overtime leave you feeling exhausted and drained with your mindset becoming increasingly influenced with negative emotions such as anxiety, fear and even depression. In this scenario it is all about timing, for the first year of your babies life you are required 110% and this is how it should be a baby needs to be close and connected to both its parents as you form the unbreakable bond that will last a life time. However, a time will come whether its 1 or 2 years later, when you could start to take back some time to refocus on you. Don't forget that old you is still there, its just not been made a priority and has been buried at the back of your hippocampus for the last 2 years (the hippocampus is the part of the brain that forms memories, in case you missed this last time, or just forgot).

Now this doesn't just relate to new parents but also those who are 100% committed to their careers, working every available hour to ensure they climb the corporate ladder as for them career progression is how they measure success in their life. Some of the unhealthiest clients I have ever worked with are city workers, bankers, lawyers and insurance brokers. The city life is surrounded by higher pressured jobs, long hours, lunches down the boozer and bags of white powder to keep them highly focused throughout the day. I have been working with one client for the last 4 years who ticks all the boxes of a typical city worker (apart from the white powder). He is an accountant and through his career has worked with celebrities, businessmen and sports professionals. He has reached the top of his profession an achievement which is highly deserved due to his selfless commitment and dedication to his career.

Due to the highly pressured environment he is surrounded by every day his own health and fitness had previously never been a priority. He was young, enthusiastic and driven he knew what he wanted, and he went for it. He came to me in his mid-40s as this lifestyle had finally crept up on him. The lack of sleep, poor diet and little exercise had created a cocktail of issues of which could no longer been shrugged off. His main objective was originally fat loss as the city life had slowly crept onto his waistline, but it did not take long to realise that there were other more concerning issues which needed addressing. His body was in a state of atrophy due to the poor diet, lack of protein and unbalanced blood sugar levels. A state of atrophy is where there is a breakdown of muscle tissue due to a lack of nutrition and little exercise.

On top of this his hormone levels were unbalanced as he was showing signs of high cortisol levels due to the weight gain around the midriff, tiredness and muscle weakness. Although cortisol has many benefits in the body, consistent high levels can be dangerous. Although cortisol has many benefits in the body, consistent high levels can be dangerous.

Cortisol is known as the stress hormone as it is generally released into the blood stream during high levels of stress. This is natures way of preparing you for a dangerous situation to increase your blood glucose levels and sharpen your focus, one role of cortisol is to prepare the body to either fight or flight from a dangerous situation. In a modern society however, we are not in a stressful state to avoid danger, we are simply dealing with societal and career-based pressures.

As a result the increase in blood glucose is not used as a form of instant energy but is left travelling around the blood stream until it is picked up and stored typically within the visceral fat cells located around the abdomen. If simply ignored this can quickly develop into obesity with an increased risk of developing hypertension and type 2 diabetes. His issues around weight gain were as a direct result of his lifestyle and consistent stress levels. By making simple improvements to his daily habits, improvement in sleep quality, basic supplementation for deficient micro nutrients and introducing a balanced diet his body fat levels will reduce. Our training sessions are vital to ensure flexibility, reverse the damage caused through the muscle atrophy and to control stress levels. His training regime is in place to ensure his body and mind remain healthy.

I cannot help but think what the long-term outcome would have been if he hadn't made that decision to change his priority list and make time to improve his health. My client now is doing well in both his career and with his health and fitness goals, he made changes to his priority list just in time. However sadly this is not the case for many people as with each year that passes their health slowly starts to deteriorate and cracks in their health start to show. But we are British, so with our stiff upper lip we just crack on, telling ourselves that the concern or discomfort will simply just pass.

Making the mindset switch to refocus on you is all about timing! Right now might not be that right time and that's fine, life is full of challenges of which are far more important than our body fat levels and so these take priority. What I do want you to do however is make a promise, not to me but to yourself, a promise that you will always be on the lookout for the right time to regain focus on yourself and to make some slight alterations to your priority list. Make a promise that when the time arises you will grab hold of it and not let it simply pass by, carpe diem (Seize the day). By making this promise you will understand that although you are not feeling at your best right now, you know that it is only for the short period of time. You now know that getting back to the person you used to be and the person you desire to be is simply a matter of timing. Just promise you will grab it when the time comes and make changes to that list. Your future self will thank you.

The dangers of letting time pass by!

The Mid-life crisis

As you get older you may hear people joke with you when you buy a new car or start going to the gym, saying that you're having a mid-life crisis that is triggering all this sudden change. Now I hope this is not the case and that you have simply made alterations to your priority list to give yourself a little more time and money when it becomes available. Sadly, this is not always the case and for some, a mid-life crisis might just be that, a crisis. The term came about in the late 19th century by an Austrian neurologist named Sigmund Freud.

He believed that during middle age, typically between the ages of 45-65, people started having thoughts that were influenced by the fear of death or the reality that they are not immortal and so sort for ways to give themselves instant gratification as compensation for the realisation of their impending doom. That was over 100 years ago and so the phrase 'mid-life crisis' has now been toned down a little. Although there has not been much substantial research into Sigmund Freuds belief the phrase 'mid-life crisis' has gained attention from popular culture in recent years. Recent studies carried out within the United States concluded that 15.5% of men and 13.3% of women felt that they had experienced the emotional roller-coaster known as a mid-life crisis and the phenomena lasted anywhere between 3 to 10 years. The research found that the emotional change was created by the sudden reality of their health and age, changes in close relationships such as with their children, and regrets over different life choices they had made with the realisation that they have little time left to make substantial changes to their life.

It would appear then that the research carried out into the reality of the 'mid-life crisis' supports the age old saying that 'its not the things they have done that people regret, it's the things they didn't do'. So why am I rambling on about all this, as I am 90% certain you are not on the verge of a mid-life crisis, the reason why, because this is all related to the decisions you make right now.

It is easy to allow time to simply slip by year after year as you tell yourself that you are ok because you know you are making a positive influence on the lives of all those closest to you. Or you are enjoying the corporate benefits your recent promotion at work has brought you along with the praise from your boss for your long-term commitment to the firm, as well as the numbers on your bank statement.

Thinking this way will eventually catch up with you, one day you will look out of the window and regret not making time for your dreams, health and aspirations and for not grabbing hold when the time passed by. I'm not saying to give up your job and spend more time with your family or to dye your hair purple and decide you want to join the circus (unless you want to), I'm talking about balance. Don't forget it's the things we don't do that we regret in later life. So, if you look back over your priority list, are you making yourself a priority? If not, why not? Through the honesty stage you came face to face with yourself, your fears, your flaws, and your desires. You know it's important to start making positive changes in your life, if right now isn't the right time it doesn't matter you will keep a look out for when it is and seize the day. If you let this time slip by then enjoy your mid-life crisis! It all starts with a simply change to your priority list.

STEP 3

Fear

The person who achieves success in life and the person who does not both started off with the same dream and the same desire, so what influenced such a difference in both outcomes? You have been through the first 2 steps to Muscling Up your Mindset you have faced your dark side and gained control of the negative chatter, you have finally altered your priority list and made a promise to yourself that you will make diet and exercise a key priority every day. So surely your squared away now and on the path to success right, wrong! There is one major roadblock that potentially stands in your way preventing you from achieving your training and fat loss goals. That roadblock is fear!!

Before we get into the detail of fear let us all understand what the word 'fear' really means. Here is one perceived definition that I found:

'Fear is a natural, powerful and primitive human emotion. It involves a universal biochemical response as well as a high individual emotional response. Fear alerts us to the presence of danger or the threat of harm whether that danger is physical or psychological. (www.verywellmind. com)

It goes without saying that everybody on earth feels fear at some points in their life, whether that be because of seeing a spider in their bedroom or as a direct threat to their life. The only part of fear that is subjective is how the individual processes the emotion of fear.

The decisions we make in life are decided deep within the frontal lobe of the brain where the thinking part seeks confirmation from the emotional to bring about a decision. Remember when I said earlier that if you allow your emotions to control your decisions you will lose yourself every time? So, it is important to listen to both the thinking and emotional parts when seeking a decision. When it comes to making decisions around self-gain there is a similar process which we all go through. In our brains the outcome of the decision is calculated by the expected value (how much you want something) by the probability that you would be able to achieve it. Research into this process goes as far back as the 17th century by a mathematician named Blaise Pascal. For a long time it was believed that representations of value and probability were being processed in the same part of the brain named the Orbital Frontal Cortex or (OFC) however recent research has shown that this decision making process is established within 2 parts, with the Ventrolateral Prefrontal Cortex or (VLPFC) also playing a key role in decision making. It is this process that makes everyones decision making ability unique. Sometimes you will find that your actions are 100% reactive and influenced by emotion, bursts of anger and an overwhelming feeling of fear would typically fall into this category. Other times you literally cannot seem to make a decision as your brain seems to be 100% clouded, although this lack of ability to focus is highly likely to be as a result of dehydration, just saying. What makes everyones decision making ability so subjective is how they allow their decisions to be influenced, whether it be through the emotional or through the thinking parts of the brain. I guarantee you know someone who always appears to be in full control of their decision making ability and able to produce a structured response no matter what situation they find themselves, an Infantry Officer in the middle of a fire fight would be typical of this mindset. I also guarantee you know someone who tends to make decisions based on how they are feeling at that particular moment, they would also be concerned about how their decision emotionally affects others, a primary school teacher may be typical of this mindset as she explains to her class the wider effects of bullying. In both examples neither is right or wrong as I said before decision making is completely subjective, and widely dependent upon the environment. The research suggests that it is how you control the influencing chatter from both the thinking and the emotional parts of the brain, that not only allows you to control your ability to make a decision, but also how you control emotions such as fear and the influence they have on your actions. To remain in full control, you should never allow decisions you make to be 100% influenced by either side. If you feel yourself becoming overwhelmed by emotion, take a step back evaluate your surroundings and formulate your decision, this is how you remain focused and in control. Do not fall victim to the negative chatter. #ITSJUSTCHATTER.

So why is all this relevant? Because fear can be your best friend or your worst enemy! You need to learn how to understand your fear, the origins of this fear and how to use this negative chatter as a powerful force of energy, powering you confidently into the gym and on the path to success. Fear it appears is very subjective and affects different people in different ways. When carrying out research into fear, many studies are also conflicting as they debate the causes of different fears and phobias and their underlining origins.

Now Muscle Up your Mindset has been written to prepare your mindset to be focused and ready to take on the huge challenge of improving your physique, health and confidence, so it makes sense to focus on the different types of fear you are likely to experience at some stage as you progress through your journey. You will be prepared to deal with this negative chatter and be armed with the ability to tame this fear and use it to your advantage. Fear will become your best friend.

The fear of judgement

The fear of judgment is probably one of the most common forms of fear many people face every day. This fear could be as simple as worrying about who you will bump into when you go shopping without your makeup on. Or being fearful about attending the gym for the first time or returning after a long break (even I get this fear). The fear of judgment is a strange emotional response as the very nature of the fear understands that in no way are you in any form of direct danger, yet we worry so much about what other people think of us, why? If your honest a fear of judgment maybe the very reason you are reading this book right now. So let's look into this fear in a little more detail so that you can recognise it and allow yourself to rise above it, as you understand it is nothing more than a little insecurity raising its head and allowing you to be negatively influenced.

There is not a person on this planet who lives their life confidently and without any form of insecurity, it is human nature to doubt ourselves and question our ability or standing within society. One fear of judgement I face every day is peoples perception on my level of success and worth. I know it does not make sense as a persons success in life is 100% subjective and is made up of so many different variables, yet I often feel as though I have not achieved enough in my life to be classed as a success when compared to others. I'll give you an example, I regularly see 2 successful young traders come into the gym together, they are younger than me, earn more money than me and so I feel a wave of disappointment come over me every time I see them, the fear of judgment creeps in as I worry about how I am perceived. Yet when thinking about it when I was their age I had just left the British Army and moved to Essex to set up my own Personal Training brand, which on paper would be text book for someone on the road to success. So, if the fear is unfounded and irrational then it can only be a representation of my own perception of myself and this is exactly what the fear of judgment is. The next time you find yourself in an environment where you feel the fear of judgment remember it is simply your own perception of yourself being projected in front of you. In order to rise above this fear you need to understand its origins and find a resolve to the insecurity which creates it.

To fully understand the fear of judgment, you also need to understand that judgement is a natural human behaviour and we all make judgments all day, every day. If you were honest and thought about it I guarantee you make judgments on more or less every person you see or come into contact with. Yet although you make these seemingly innocent judgments on people every day, you still hold such a fear of being judged yourself. If I was to ask you about some of the people you saw the last time you were in a supermarket you would probably struggle. No doubt at the time you made innocent judgments about people as you were walking round, because its human nature to do so. However as quickly as you judged a person, you forget about it and carry on with your life because that's what we do.

It is through this process that we decide where we fit in within society and amongst our peers and work colleagues, it's an essential process to allow us to build meaningful relationships, some which will last a life time. So although the fear of judgment is one of the most common forms of fear, it's also one in which we can easily overcome. Trying to be liked by every person we meet is exhausting and is actually bad for your health as you portray yourself in a way you feel is socially acceptable. By simply being yourself not only will you release yourself from the burden of judgment fear, but people will become drawn to your positivity. Some people will judge you, of course they will its human nature to do so but these people will in no way play any part in your life, so it doesn't matter. What does matter are those that are drawn to you, those that have judged you positively and as a result a new relationship is born. This fear is literally holding you back from stepping outside of your comfort zone and achieving success. Allowing yourself to overcome your fear of being judged by others is a mindset challenge you will need to understand and in time overcome, you could call this process Muscling Up your Mindset.

The fear of Conflict.

When you look into the origins of people who you perceive to have achieved a level of success in their life, there always tends to be one similar characteristic and that is the level of support they had around them from friends, family and mentors. Right now you are about to embark on a very challenging yet positive journey and one which will result in making changes to what was your daily routine, changes which are designed to improve your life in all aspects.

As humans we are often intrinsically wired to be resistant to any form of change from our daily routine also known as our comfort zone, this can result in conflict from those closest to you. Before beginning this journey it is important to recognise any fear of conflict that you currently have deep within your negative mindset as this will result in the voice of negativity influencing certain decisions you need to make, ultimately resulting in you dropping out from this process. A fear of conflict can be present in many different forms, worrying about how other people will react to any changes that you make. Worrying about any negativity that might come your way from those closest to you or arguments around your time committed to training and dietary choices at mealtimes. These are all common fears that clients have at the start of their journey as they begin to impose a new regime, one that is different from the norm. I can completely understand why a new client may have this fear of conflict within their own home as through doing something positive for themselves, conflict has arisen, disrupting the peace at home. If this is a fear you currently have before starting this program then please understand that you are taking a positive step forward to help benefit your life and your health because no one else is going to do this for you. I commend you for having the confidence and bravery to do so, so please do not let anyone knock you down especially not those closest to you. As I mentioned earlier everyone walking this planet has insecurities and at times emotional responses cause their insecurities to be projected in front of them. When a person starts to take positive and proactive steps in their life, they will always come across confrontation from individuals who feel threatened, judged and envious due to their own portrayal of themselves as a result of their insecurities.

Believe me when I say this type of negativity is only going to drag you down especially if you feel this confrontation and emotional response to your life changes is going to come from someone closest to you. Is this a situation you are fearful off? If not skip this chapter and move on, if it is then here is my advice on how to move forward.

1. Get them on side: Before you start this journey, you need to have a strong support network around you to help motivate and support your life changes. So, one of the first challenges you will have is to get your closest family members on side, explain to them what you are doing and the reasons why. If your partner starts to worry that your newly found confidence and determination to improve your physique is a result of a desire to attract others then reassure them that it's not and that you are simply doing this for you. Unless it is to attract others in which case crack on. Once your partner is on side your life will become so much easier and you can start to implement the required changes.

2. Make plans with your partner: One of the biggest causes of conflict is meal times, the client is managing their calorie intake and so their meals need to be managed however their partner just wants a curry on a Saturday night, conflict straight away. So, the way to avoid this is to plan your weekly meals in advance with your partner so that they feel they still have a say in what food you are both cooking. If your clever with your weekly calorie management, you may even be able to fit in a curry on a Saturday night which I am sure you will both enjoy.

3.   Be firm with your regime: The worst thing you could do when your partner applies a little bit of pressure is to back down. The very process of you going against your new regime will highlight to your partner that it cannot be that important and so the same conflict will happen again and again. Stay firm on your approach to your new regime and ensure your partner is aware that there is little negotiation due to how important this process is to you. Over time your partner will start to accept this as the new norm and you never know they may even start to join in with you in which case well done you have just made an very positive impact on someone very close to you, well done.

4.   If none of the above works and you continue to get conflict at home despite all attempts to get them on-board in supporting you. Then sorry to be brutally honest but you may need to get a new partner. This whole process is to help improve your life and so I am here to help you, not them. If this is the brutal reality of your situation then steps may need to be made to allow you to live a life full of happiness and positivity, because that is what you deserve.

The fear of failure.

Before we go into the detail of why we have a fear of failure, let's try and understand what your perception of failure really is as failure especially a fear of failure is very subjective and differs from person to person. So, for a minute please stop reading this book and think about what areas of your life are you afraid of failing in, and then answer the questions below, even write them down if it helps:

Where do you think those fears have come from?

_____

Has this fear negatively affected the outcome of something positive in your life previously?

_____

Do you feel as though you are able to overcome this fear of failure?

_____

The fear of failure also known as 'atychiphobia' is something I am all too familiar with and still battle to this day. Even writing this book right now the voice of negativity is in the back of mind telling me that no one is going to find any of this interesting or remotely useful. However it's 12:15pm on Friday 13th November 2020 and I am finally determined to prove to myself that I can be more, achieve more and help you to do the same. So, what is the definition of a 'fear of failure'? Here is one definition I found which for me perfectly fits its characteristics.

'The Fear of Failure is when we allow that fear to stop us doing the things that can move us forward to achieve our goals'. www.MindTools.com (1st page of Google I know)

This is exactly how I view the fear of failure which haunts many decisions I have made in my past as well as my present and no doubt my future. To me the fear of failure is the annoying voice of negativity which lingers at the back of my mind and raises its head every time I attempt to step outside of my comfort zone and move forward. As you learnt in the earlier stages of this book every decision we make in life are influenced by the voice of negativity and the voice of positivity, which voice you choose to listen to ultimately determines the overall outcome, this is no different. So, let us look at this fear through a positive mindset and understand it for what it is. Atychiphobia is exactly what the name suggests, it is a phobia! Let's look at the definition of a phobia:

'Phobias are irrational fears relating to specific objects or situations. Atychiphobia is an irrational fear of failing'.

The key word here is 'irrational' as fear itself does not exist, you cannot physically see it, touch or feel it. Fear is simply an evolutional survival mechanism allowing us to foresee danger before it occurs. Fear is your own imagination projecting your worst-case scenario in front of you. Now for many people the fear of failure comes from being a perfectionist, especially in areas of your life where you want to succeed such as your career or your marriage. Before taking any positive steps forward and outside of your safe zone you will always carry out a subconscious risk assessment of all possible threats, dangers and possible outcomes. Now for me I will always start off with wild possible outcomes when I begin any new project, for example when I started writing this book in my head it was going to be a Times best seller and be proudly displayed as you walk into Waterstones. This positivity never lasts long as the risk assessment is carried out in my mind I start to run through all other possible outcomes, with the worst being this becomes yet another document which sits on my laptop never to be seen or read by anyone. Now the positive thinker will carry out their risk assessment, acknowledge that is a potential outcome and focus on the original highly positive result. For the perfectionist however this is rarely the case as we can easily become consumed by the fear of the latter outcome and the disappointment failure would bring. So, the overall outcome is we down tools accept the disappointment failure would bring would be too much to handle and stay wrapped up within our safety blanket glued to our current existence.

Not everyone will experience this fear in the same way however, as with most phobias there is a scale from mild to severe. A mild phobia would mean you see the failed outcome, understand it is a possibility but push passed this to form a positive result. A more severe phobia will result in other aspects of your life becoming affected as this fear starts affecting your work, social and home life. The problem with more severe cases of Atychiphobia is you are almost creating your own reality. By becoming so immersed in the fear of a failed outcome you sub-consciously start to sabotage any positive efforts you could be making, which is only going to end in a negative result.

Let's relate this to a fat loss scenario.

You are a female in your late 20's, your looking to reduce your body fat as you have noticed your clothes are starting to become a lot tighter. Your confidence has been knocked as you fear you may need to go up a dress size and worry about how you may be judged by others. So you join a local slimming club, purchase their cook books and start carrying out their regime. You have been restricting yourself from foods you enjoy as they are classed as sins and have been trying so hard to be good and achieve your weekly goals. In the back of your mind you know that if this diet does not work the end result will be you having to go up a dress size and require a new wardrobe. This negative outcome then starts to manifest itself into your sub-conscious mindset as you understand this could realistically be the outcome, and so a fear of failure starts to creep in.

Three weeks later you weigh yourself again, to find the weight has gone up despite all your restrictions and best efforts. That voice of negativity starts influencing your mindset telling you that you're never going to be thin again and your destined for a life as an over weight whale. Your action on the back of this is you go home, buy a bottle of wine and some chocolate and spend the night on the sofa. You wake up the next day completely demotivated, scrap the diet and return back to your previous dietary habits.

Now the reason for the weight gain had nothing to do with the fact you had gained body fat. You were simply starting the luteal phase of your menstrual cycle and so that gain on the scales was due to an increase in water retention because of an oestrogen surge. If you had continued your diet regime for another week you would have stepped back on the scales and chances are would have seen a decrease in around 2lbs in body weight. In this example the fear of failure sabotaged all the positive steps that had been made in the first 3 weeks. The voice of negativity had influenced the decisions and so the result was the worst-case scenario, relapse and probably weight gain.

I really do not want this for you, hence why I have added this section into the book.

If you do suffer from a fear of failure, please do not be too hard on yourself as chances are it stems from a past experience which has either happened to you or someone close to you. After carrying out further research into the fear of failure I found the phobia to be as a result of three scenarios;

1.   You have past experience where you've failed, especially if the situation was traumatic or the result was important such as missing out on a job.

2.   You have learnt to fear failing through different situations.

3.   You are a perfectionist

Now for me I know exactly where my fear of failure comes from as I take myself right back to the moment I was sat on my bed with my head in my hands, I had arrived back from Lichfield after failing my Army career. This experience taught me a lot, and I would even go as far as to say it is what fuels my desire and determination to be successful today so in a way, I am thankful for the life lesson and it wasn't long before I was back in green skin (Army uniform). Understanding what the underlying causes are for your fear of failure will help you to understand that its ok to be fearful, as actually the fear is only there to protect you from further disappointment. From this moment however what you need to do, is to understand the fear for what it is. It is nothing more than an irrational phobia, it is simply the voice of negativity trying to keep you wrapped up within your safe zone. Understand that the worst-case scenario is a possible outcome, but also remember you ultimately decide if the outcome is positive or not. By repeatedly concerning yourself with the worst-case scenario you will sabotaging any positive steps you could be making. You decide if the outcome is positive or negative and after Muscling Up your Mindset you no longer have a choice as after reading this book every decision you make will be a positive step forward.

STEP 4

Ownership

So far we have explored the different psychological challenges you face every day and learnt how to overcome these to create the best possible outcome. You have taken time to look deeper into your mindset and discover what you desire in your life. You have reviewed your priority list and leant that by making simple changes to your daily habits incredible results can be achieved. Now it's time to take command of your own destiny, it's time for you to take ownership of your life, the challenges that are faced every day and the positivity of their outcome. One of the hardest realities of life is understanding that you are in full control of every outcome you are presented with. Even when the outcome of the event is out of your hands, how you move forward is 100% in your control as you decide to accept this outcome positively or negatively before you move on. The question is are you able to accept the reality of the situations presented to you? Or do you take the easy route out and play the victim card pushing blame for the outcome into another direction or onto another person.

When it comes to taking the positive step forward and deciding to improve your health and fitness, it is vital that you prepare yourself psychologically before you begin, hence why you are reading this book right now. The 5 steps you are taking to Muscling Up your Mindset are to allow you to understand the deeper motivation behind your desire for change and to understand that you are in full control over the outcome and the positive influence this change can have in all aspects of your life.

As mentioned earlier within this book 50% of people who join the gym leave within just 6 months. Now I know there are many different variables which effect a persons decision to drop out of this process and I do not mean to throw out a sweeping statement. That said if you were to take full ownership of your decisions and understand your desire and drive behind the change, then your motivation will insure that you are part of the 50% of people who adopt a new healthier and more active life, the ownness is on you to take full ownership of this process. Not many people know this but apart from being an online trainer, I also manage the fitness products within 3 health clubs in London, working with Group Exercise Instructors, Fitness Motivators and Personal Trainers to deliver an unbeatable product which encourages people to retain at the club and adopt a healthier lifestyle.

By far the most common reason we see for membership cancellations is the fact they have no time. I always find this excuse interesting because you have 24 hours in every day and have 24-hour gyms, meaning you can train at literally any time you have available. However, what this excuse tells me straight away is that a lack of time is not the issue, what the 'I have no time' excuse really means is 'it's not a priority'. That's fine but you need to take ownership of the fact you decide what your top priorities are every day and if becoming fitter and healthier is not one of them you will never be in the right mindset to adopt the daily habits required. By using the 'no time' excuse, you have actively decided not to continue with the process so need to take ownership of that decision and realise it was yours to make. What we choose to do with the hours given to us every day is one of the most important decisions we make as it determines the direction and success of our life.

As a father, husband, business owner and a Contract Fitness Manager I have little time for myself, so have a degree of sympathy for those who are literally struggling to find time for personal growth. That said there are 24 hours in a day, not simply the typical 15 hours a person tends to be awake. So, for me I use unsociable hours to get things that I need done and have highlighted this at several points in the book. Now for example its 5:08am I have just changed my little boy's nappy and given him a bottle, this gives me about another 1:30 hours to crack on with required tasks, such as writing this book. Take ownership of the hours available to you in the day and how you wish to use them, like I said this is the biggest decision you have to make every day, so use it wisely.

How often you push blame for your actions depends on what's known as your 'Locus of Control' more on this later. So, let us look at some other common excuses we make in order to deflect responsibilities for our failures. Have a look through these and see how many you may find yourself occasionally saying:

- *I have always been over-weight it is a genetic trait in our family.*
- *It is too cold to do any exercise today I will start tomorrow*
- *It is too late to do any exercise now I will start again Monday*
- *I am over the age of 40 I am too old to change my health and fitness.*
- *It is not my fault I'm often late for work, it's due to traffic.*
- *I will not get a promotion at work because my boss does not like me.*

Now I'll be honest, the traffic excuse I have definitely said a couple of times in my life, but let's look at how a simple lack of ownership around your work commitment can have a knock-on effect. The traffic excuse is commonly used within every workplace, in many cases instead of the traffic being the direct reason for the lateness it becomes an acceptable excuse to justify poor work commitment and employee organisation. The second excuse, ' I won't get promoted at work because my boss doesn't like me', looking at this example the individual wouldn't get promoted at work because they were typically late and so yes their boss did not like them but this was due to their own actions. For this to change the employee would need to take ownership of their reputation and understand why their employer has concerns. It now becomes the employee's responsibility to change this perception to progress their career. The employee found an acceptable excuse to justify their lack of organisation and did not realise that this then resulted in a poor reputation. They did not get promoted because their boss did not like them, they didn't get promoted because they were unreliable. For the employee it was much easier to believe they didn't get promoted because their boss did not like them, as opposed to accepting the fact they have not been promoted due to their own failures towards their work commitment.

Playing the victim card and blaming external factors for our circumstances is almost habit for many people however up until now this is not their fault. We are growing up within a society that from a young age is reaffirming to us that the world is a dangerous and unjust place. When we are a child our parents and teachers are always telling us not to touch this or that and to walk and not run.

We are told this is dangerous and that is hot and have to wash our hands after coming into contact with the smallest amount of mycobacteria. We are being told repeatedly 'be careful, be careful, BE CAREFUL' by the responsible people closest to us, reaffirming once again the world is full of danger. This is more relevant now than ever as currently we cannot step outside of our homes without wearing a face covering or handle food shopping without wearing latex gloves. We are being told to stay in our homes and only leave when necessary for items such as food or medication. All over the TV news channels are reporting the number of deaths that are occurring and how a virus is spreading round the country faster than I can type this sentence. As a result, fully grown adults are scared to leave their homes due to the whole world telling them to 'be careful' and once again reaffirming that the world is a dangerous place. Many people are feeling overwhelmed by the current complexity of modern life and are feeling unsure as to their role and responsibility within it. Right now, there has never been a more important time to step back and take a moment for self-reflection. It is important you take ownership of your current situation and to no longer shift blame in other directions. Not only can your physical health be affected by your lack of responsibility, but your mental and emotional health can also be at risk. Thankfully like all bad habits, this negative way of thinking can be reversed and you can start to regain ownership of your life.

Attack of the Locus

How we respond to the different situations presented to us every day is influenced by many different variables such as age, personality, upbringing, and environment.

However how we view our environment and all the positivity and negativity included within it all depends on what is known as 'Locus of Control', I can literally hear you saying what the hell is that? Here is the definition:

'Locus of control is the degree to which people believe that they, as opposed to external forces (beyond their influence), have control over the outcome of events in their lives'. Wikipedia

So let's bring this back to you and see which of the 2 options below are closer to your personality:

Internal Locus of Control

If you have an internal locus of control you are more internally aware of your actions and take ownership of the decisions you make every day. You work hard for the things you want in life and take ownership of the outcome of your decisions. You prioritise your daily tasks based upon what is most important to you.

External Locus of Control

If you have an external Locus of Control then you are far more likely to deflect responsibility for your actions and push blame for the outcome. You often make excuses for your failures and blame external factors or other people for the negative outcome. You are more prone to anxiety and struggle to handle stressful situations. As a result, you are less likely to strive for what you want out of life as you remain wrapped up safely within your comfort zone.

Now let's Muscle Up your Mindset and start to make real change, here is what you need to do to internalise your locus:

1. Notice your tendency to push blame: Think back to our traffic example, now be honest and ask yourself how often your push blame for your actions in other directions? Do you take ownership of situations and be honest about you role in the outcome? If you tend to avoid taking responsibility, then start to take notice of how often this occurs and manage accordingly.

2. Focus on finding a solution: In the earlier stages of this book I asked you to think about what it really is that your looking to achieve through this process and dig deep, examples include improving your health, wealth, confidence or maybe all 3. From now on you are always going to find a way around the hurdles that stand in the way of your success, no matter what those hurdles are. You will take full responsibility of these hurdles as they are yours and yours only, face them, acknowledge them, and then find a solution around them.

3. Start saying I choose....: Change the way you view the decisions you make every day, even when you feel like you're not making a decision you are, as you are actively deciding not to approach the issue pro actively. When you are setting yourself targets for the day instead of saying, 'I need to' or 'I must' start saying 'I choose to', for example 'I choose to take the dog for a walk', instead of negatively saying ' I must take the dog for a walk'. Similarly, if you say to yourself, 'I'm too tired to go to the gym', start saying 'I choose not to go to the gym'.

This simple change in language psychologically means you are taking full ownership of all the decisions you are making. As a result, you are not able to push blame in other directions and accept full responsibility of the outcome. This way you are subconsciously going to be looking to create more positive outcomes from the decisions you make, as after all it is 100% in your control. You will be amazed how much positivity is created by this simple change alone.

4. Do something every day that scares you: I was told this as a child and for some reason it has always stuck with me, although back then I had no idea what it meant. By doing something every day that scares you, reaffirms to you that the world is not as dangerous as our environment is trying to convince us it is. To achieve personal growth in life, it often requires you to step outside of your comfort zone and into the unknown. As you have learnt already within this book, the very process of doing so is fuel for the negative mindset which will attempt with vigour to discourage you. By allowing yourself to become uncomfortable every day improves how confident you feel when outside your area of safety. This will help to improve irrational fears such as the fear of judgment and as a result start to improve your confidence in handling different uncomfortable situations.

Here are some simple ways you can step outside of your comfort zone:

1. Sit on a bench and ask a stranger for the time.
2. Go to a social environment on your own such as a restaurant or the cinema
3. Confidently take selfies in public
4. Say hello to a stranger as you walk past them.
5. Give someone a compliment unexpectedly.
6. Attend a gym class on your own
7. Spend some time away from your phone, leave it at home when you go out.
8. If your single then be brave to approach people and ask for a number

From today I want you to make a promise to yourself that you will stop pushing blame for the decisions and actions you make in other directions. Once you take ownership of all the variables involved within your daily life you will be in a better position to consider how to respond to the challenges presented to you. Hold yourself responsible and you will rethink your approach. Suddenly you will become more proactive, dependable, and successful this reputation can only have positive effects in all aspects of your life. So be brave, be confident and remember you are in full control.

STEP 5

Consistency

Every single one us has the power to be more and achieve more in our lives. We come up with amazing ideas and take great leaps of faith into the unknown, all with the aim to improve the happiness and positivity of our life. However sadly it is far more common for these ideas to slowly die as the initial hype settles down and the reality of what is required to be successful soaks in. Let us be honest, for most people consistency is an impossible hurdle to overcome. It ultimately results in that once great idea becoming another failed attempt, achieving nothing more than to reaffirm to you that you are incapable of success. It is no wonder so many people are struggling from forms of anxiety and even depression. This was one of the reasons I wanted to write this short book, as I know exactly how it feels to be a failure in your own mind as you fail to achieve the outcome you were so excited about just weeks earlier. If you relate to this in any way, then please this stops now! I hope you have learnt through reading this book that you have the power to decide the outcome of the decisions you make. It all starts with a positive mindset and the understanding that the key to success lies with the understanding of the following 3 statements:

The first statement I want you to remember, 'Nothing worth having comes easy', this is true in all aspects of life and improving your health and fitness is no different, this does come with good news however.

After completing this book, you will move onto the first section of your 'Progress Tracker' and begin learning the daily habits that need to be adopted in order to achieve the positive outcome you seek.

You will learn the reasoning behind all the life changes you need to adopt and the positive effects they will have every day. The good news is once you have completed this section you will feel more confident than ever that success is simply a matter of time. The intrinsic motivation to get started will be burning deep within you, and this is exactly where you need to be as you learn the process is quite simple. Nothing worth having comes easy and so the hard part is the fact the outcome is 100% in your control and this can be a bitter pill to swallow if the outcome is not positive (but that won't happen, so don't worry). Success requires the consistent adoption of the required daily habits as not only are they in place for you to be successful short term but also so that the body fat never returns, resulting in long term, sustainable success. You will start to view your body composition change as you did your virginity, once its gone its gone and you never have to worry about it again. What happens after this is the exciting part as improving your body confidence is simply just the start. Once you get a taste of how incredibly good success feels you are going to want more, I promise you! This leads to an intrinsic desire to be achieve in all aspects of your life and for me this is how you measure real success. I am excited for you, as I know you are on the cusp of a new adventure and one I am proud to have had a very small part in. Right now is a very exciting and positive time in your life, but just remember to give yourself time and remember nothing worth having comes easy but you will be armed with a focused and determined mindset so any challenges you face will be hurdled as a positive mindset conquers all.

The second statement I want you to remember is 'Good things come to those who wait', and I'm not talking about drinking Guinness, although you do have to wait ages at the bar for that bad boy. As mentioned previously in this book I need you to be prepared to play the long game. The process you are about to go through either with me or on your own is not simply a quick fix to reduce your body fat. It is a lifelong journey of striving every day to be a better person than you were the day before. You achieve this by setting yourself daily habits and ticking them off at the end of the day. This simple little habit alone can generate immense pride, when you've finished a hard day and notice you have still achieved everything you set out to when you woke up, gives you a real internal sense of achievement. These daily challenges will change as you grow and develop and this is a good thing as it shows you have been confident enough to step outside of your comfort zone and accept an element of risk. Just remember by tackling a challenging situation with a positive mindset can only create a positive result, if you do this day in day out then this is where a fulfilled and happy life exists. Right now, you have to understand that this does not happen overnight, just as real success can't be achieved by just simply dropping a few lbs and buying some new clothes. What you are doing right now is allowing positive change to influence your life, adopt my mantra, and you will be amazed how much life can offer you. For me right now in the UK we are in the middle of our second lockdown and this means I have a little more free time, all be it not a great deal as my little boy keeps me more than busy.

So as with the rising of a new day comes a new challenge and mine right now is to complete this book so that I can send it to print and add it to my other products, which when combined have the ability to really change a persons life, or at least make a difference. All you must do right now, is complete the daily tasks set with a positive attitude, face any challenge head on and then remain patient, success comes from consistency.

The third statement I want you to remember is, 'It all starts with you', I love this saying, it was first introduced to me while listening to an audio book by ex Special Forces Operator Ant Middleton, an individual who I can safely say has had a profound and positive influence on my mindset and determination to achieve. What I like most about this saying is its pure honesty, it is not a sexy or uplifting quote, it simply reminds you that every decision you make in life was made by you. It reminds you that the direction your life is heading, is because of your acknowledgement of the influencing factors which resulted in your chosen decision. If you feel as though your life is heading down a steep spiral then it is 100% down to you to accept your reality and put in place the required daily habits to improve the positivity of your environment. It all starts with you, and the will power to approach daily challenges with a positive mindset. However you are reading this book right now so I can only assume that this is not really relevant for you, you seized an opportunity as you saw the value this process could bring to your life, you made a decision which can only create a positive result, for this I commend you.

At some point you sat on the sofa and thought I want to make a positive change to my life, reduce my body fat and build my confidence. There have been thousands of successful people who have been sat in the same seat you are right now, they faced the challenges and rose triumphant. There have also been thousands of people who have been sat in the same seat you are right now and failed, the only difference being a dent in their bank balance and their self-esteem. The only variable that separates the 2 outcomes is the mindset of the person taking on the challenge. The person that says they will succeed and the person that says they will fail are both right as they have already decided their outcome. Remember it all starts with you! Make the decision to allow positive change to happen, complete the daily tasks required with a positive mindset and be consistent. This is the recipe of success; this is how you Muscle Up your Mindset.

The time for action is now!

If you are reading this now then we have just been through an incredible journey together, we have been through the lowest moments in our lives and taken time to understand the person staring back at us in the mirror. This process has bonded us as we start to form an unbreakable team, I hope you are now ready to move onto the next phase and prepare to take action. Through reading this book you have learnt that you hold all the power in deciding the outcome of this process, however you are not facing this challenge on your own, I am here with you. Within this book I have been with you in spirit but believe me that I had you in mind as I made my way through each section. My objective was to present you with as many solutions as possible to create the best possible outcome.

A great superhero once said;

'With great power comes great responsibility' Spiderman – The Peter Parker principle.

The next section of this book allows you to take note on all the required actions from Muscle Up your Mindset. As with all decisions within this book the responsibility to action all you have learnt through parts 1 and 2 is down to you, take ownership of this opportunity. I have kept this book reasonably short for a reason, I wanted you to be able to absorb all the information I presented you with and allow you to confidently take action.

I know from past experience many books are purchased with all the intention in the world to complete. However due to greater priorities and little time, they end up on the shelf gathering dust next to diet books from an array of different chefs and authors, some half read and others a single page has never been turned.

Reading a book and absorbing the knowledge is great short term as seeds are planted and hopefully daily habits are adopted. But overtime information is forgotten and once scheduled changes are nothing more than reminders on a phone. So it is important that all the desired outcomes, emotions felt and required changes to your daily habits are written down and referred to regularly throughout your journey to allow you to see exactly how far you have come. One of the key lessons within this book is the importance of intrinsic motivation. Through reading parts 1 and 2 of this book you now know this is achieved through clear understanding of your motivating factors and desired outcomes. What also aids intrinsic motivation is clearly seeing the results of all your hard work and the positive changes you have made to your life. By putting pen to paper allows you to document the exact details of your current mindset and the objectives you are setting out to achieve, thus giving you an action plan to crack on with and a standard to hit.

So right now, I want you to stop reading and complete the questions on the next page. These questions will outline your overall training objectives and the motivating factors behind them, so please be as detailed as you like......

MUSCLE UP YOUR MINDSET

The pen is mightier than the sword, this saying is no truer than right now as it's time for you to bare all. Complete the questions below and start to piece together your action plan:

Are you ready to 100% commit to this process?

YES   **NO**   **NOT YET**

Has there been a particular event in your life that still influences decisions you make today?

_____

_____

_____

_____

Are you able to process this memory and take away the lessons you have learnt?

YES   **NO**   **NOT YET**

What are your desired outcomes from this process?

1. _____

2. _____

3. _____

Why are these desired changes important to you?

1. _____

_____

2. _____

_____

3. _____

_____

How will achieving these desired outcomes influence other aspects of your life?

1. _____

_____

2. _____

_____

3. _____

_____

List your top 5 daily priorities at this moment in your life:

1. _____

2. _____

3. _____

4. _____

5. _____

Are you still ready to 100% commit to this process?

YES   **NO**   **NOT YET**

What are your biggest fears relating to this process?

_____

_____

_____

_____

Are you able to remain in control of these fears as you
understand this is negativity attempting to influence
your decisions?

YES   **NO**   **NOT YET**

Do you understand that success is 100% in your control
and you are able to take ownership of the outcome and
all associated decisions you make?

YES   **NO**   **NOT YET**

You understand this process is not a quick fix and that right now you are changing your life. You are committed to making the required alterations to your daily habits in order to achieve your desired outcomes.

YES **NO** **NOT YET**

Are you willing to make a promise to yourself that you will step outside of your comfort zone and never look back?

YES **NO** **NOT YET**

You are an Inspiration

If the answers to all these questions have been positive then congratulations, you have just Muscled Up your Mindset. I want to thank you so much for staying with me through the whole of this book as you experienced some of the most memorable moments of my life and understood the lessons they have taught me. I am so excited to see all the positive changes you are about to make in your own life and the amazing results these changes will bring, you really are an inspiration. I want to finish this part of the book with 2 quotes:

'Nothing is impossible, the word itself says I'm Possible'.
Audrey Hepburn

'Once your mindset changes, everything on the outside changes with it' Steve Maraboli

PART 3

Moving on to the next stage!

So what happens now? Right now, psychologically you are 100% ready to begin this process, I would even say you have been through the hardest phase, so well done! It's time for you to move onto the education phase, you are ready to adopt positive change into your life and so it is important from day 1 that you adopt the correct daily habits, after all:

'You are a walking representation of your daily habits'.

Understanding all aspects of the process you are about to begin is vital to achieve your desired outcomes with long term results. The fitness industry is FULL of 'so called' gurus misinforming you about how success is achieved to either plug a commission code or sell their services. If the key to success lies within your daily habits then it is vital that the correct habits are adopted from day 1, and here is the reason why:

'It can take anywhere from 18 to 254 days for a person to form a new habit and an average of 66 days for a new behaviour to become automatic' (www.Healthline.com)

The biggest mistake you can make at this point right now is to start implementing the wrong changes, it can literally add months before you gain sustainable results. But do not worry I have you covered, in Part 3 you move over to my next book, congratulations you have been promoted to my 'Progress Tracker'.

With the 'Progress Tracker' you will learn everything you need to know about all the variables effecting successful fat loss and muscular hypertrophy. I will go into detail on the mechanisms within the body which create fat loss and show you how to structure your calorie intake to ensure you are either in a calorie deficit or surplus depending on your desired outcomes. I will make supplementation simple and explain what supplements are worth taking and what are not. But most importantly I will introduce you to the daily habits you need to adopt into your daily routine and the reasons why they are so important.

I've still got your back!

At the start of this book I promised you I would be with you all the way through your first 12 weeks, so the support does not end there, I've still got you covered!

After completing the education phase of the 'Progress Tracker' you will then move onto the 'Action' phase as you start to put all you have learnt into practise. If you haven't already done so now is the perfect time to head over to www.JamesRobertson.fitness and grab hold of your first 12 week progressive training program. The 'Progress Tracker' is exactly as the name suggest, it is there as a tool to allow you to manage all your required daily habits. There is a page for every day which you will need to complete, you will record all the variables which effect your results including; calories, sleep, hydration, exercise, daily steps, stress levels....

Please remember the following statement;

'You can't change what you don't manage', so staying in control of all effecting variables is vital every day, or at least for the first 66 days before they become automatic.

This is now the end of the book, but the beginning of a new and exciting chapter in your life. Thank you for joining me through this journey it has been a pleasure, however this is not where our journey ends. Now I need you to close this chapter in your life by closing this book and open a new chapter of your life by opening the page to my 'Progress Tracker'.

So if you're ready, let's begin......

Printed in Great Britain
by Amazon

77928564R00069